The Pregnancy Journey through Yoga

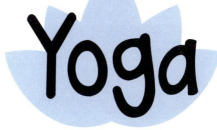

Written by Francisco
Photography by Dan Knudson Productions
Book Design by Yasmin Obradovich

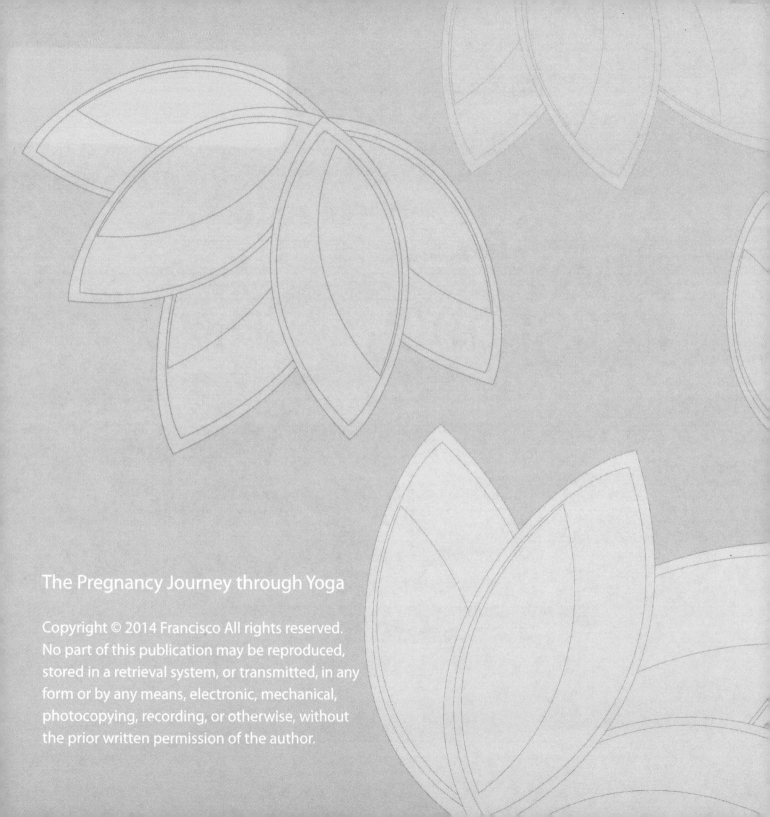

The Pregnancy Journey through Yoga

Copyright © 2014 Francisco All rights reserved. No part of this publication may be reproduced, stored in a retrieval system, or transmitted, in any form or by any means, electronic, mechanical, photocopying, recording, or otherwise, without the prior written permission of the author.

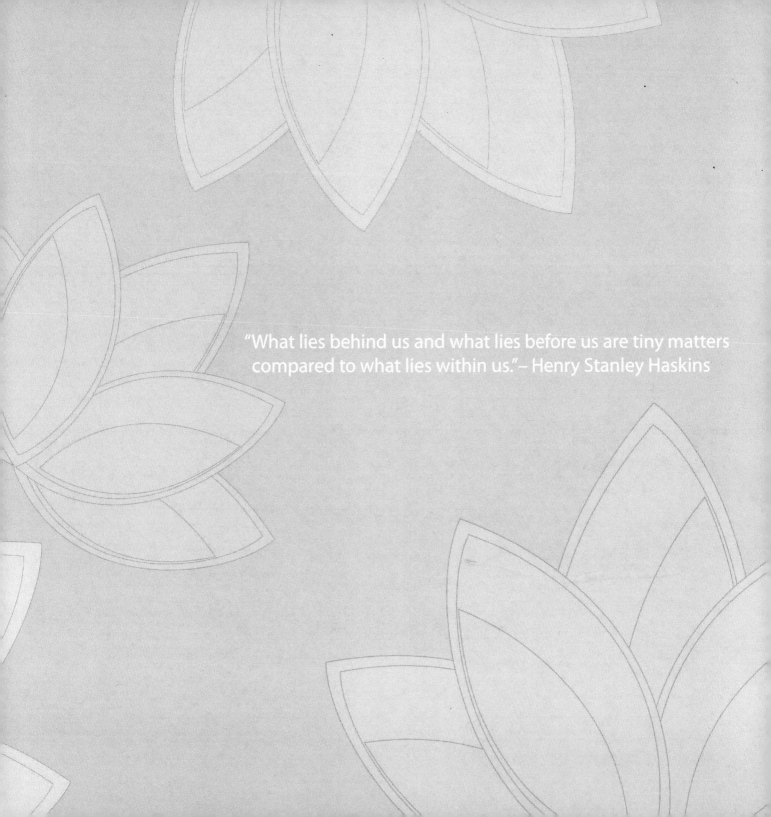

"What lies behind us and what lies before us are tiny matters compared to what lies within us." – Henry Stanley Haskins

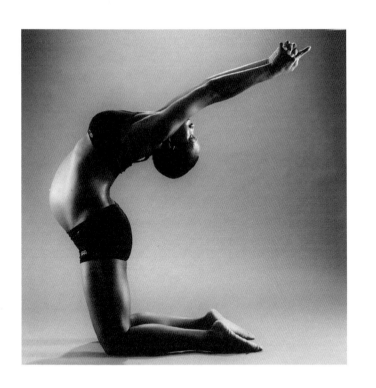
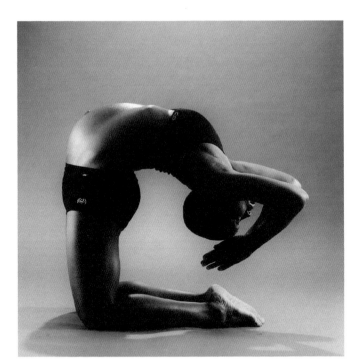
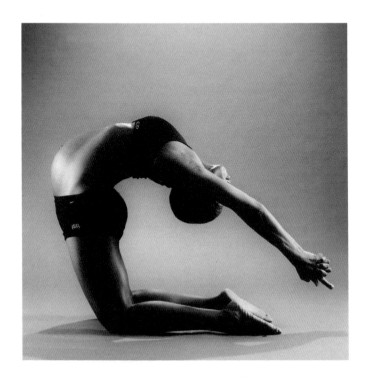
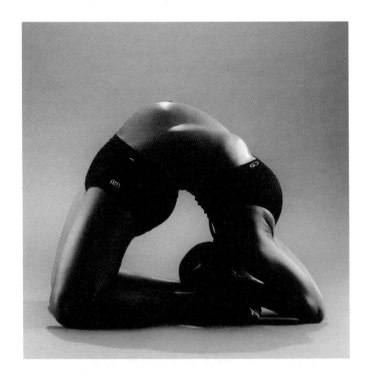

Index

Foreward	7
Introducion	8
Lisa Richards	14
Paulina Villanez - Arvizu	26
Julie Eberle Pelaz	34
Jordin Murphree	44
Chau Kei Ngai	54
Lara Carey	64
Sonja Wyche	76
Emily Carpenter	88
Thank You	106

Foreword

When my dear friend Francisco asked me to write a forward for his inspiring book "The Pregnancy Journey Through Yoga," I was both honored and humbled. To write in the company of such amazing women who have faced their pregnancy and delivery with such strength and love is such a gif. I have experienced this both as a mother and a clinician.

As a women's health Physiotherapist for the last 10 plus years, I have cared for many inspiring mothers, both during and after their pregnancies. My work in the clinic always emphasized helping women remain mobile, functional & active throughout their pregnancy, while respecting gentle medical precautions to keep both mother and baby safe. My greatest advice for safety during pregnancy is to "follow your instinct for what your body and baby need." Francisco has captured this premise with such perfection.

This book is an illustrative homage to the gift of movement that all mothers can share with their babies from conception, through childhood and into adulthood. Yoga is a perfect personification of the connection between intuition, beauty, movement/mobility and self awareness/connection. I recommend prenatal yoga to all of the mothers I care for as a lovely way to connect with their inner self, with their physical bodies (through movement and awareness) and with their babies developing within. Listening to their own perfect instincts is central to the yoga teachings, and the most organic way to stay moving throughout pregnancy.

in love, in intuition, in movement,

Nicole M Dority, DPT, MSPT, OCS
Women's Health Physiotherapist, Denver, Colorado
Fellow yogi and mother

Introduction

The moments leading up to birth have a huge impact on both mother and child. What a woman goes through—her habits, her emotions, what she consumes, and her physical activities—all have an impact on the child she is carrying. For her child, a mother is a vehicle into this life. We should take care of our mothers, and our mothers should take care of us; in this union of being in the womb, we are celebrating life.

In this book, you will read about the experiences of yoga mommas. You will also see brilliant images of these women taking care of themselves in a way that our modern world is beginning to appreciate more and more. Today, we are starting to understand that a woman's body is instinctively equipped to care for her child. By taking care of her body, she can begin to nurture her child before the actual birth.

Today, as yoga is being popularized in the West, women are realizing what a tremendous impact yoga practice can have on their pregnancy. I am amazed by the courageous paths taken by these mamas. It is important to share their stories with other women embarking on similar paths.

When a pregnant woman first came to a yoga class I was teaching, I was at a loss for words. I had no idea how to be of assistance to her or how to answer her questions. I began to ask my sister questions about her four pregnancies, and I studied the anatomy of a woman during pregnancy. Slowly, I informed myself about posture modifications for pregnant women.

As I learned how to assist them, I became more and more inspired by women who decided to continue their yoga practice during pregnancy. Many had to do so against doctors' advice. Instead, they relied on what their intuition told them was best.

That intuition—that mind and body connection they established through their yoga practice—became invaluable as they nurtured the life growing inside. With the aid of their yoga practice, they were able to remain healthy during pregnancy and adjust to this amazing change.

They were also able to achieve natural childbirth at a time when Cesarean sections were very popular. These women recovered from childbirth more rapidly and retained their level of fitness and sense of well being after giving birth. In order to educate others, it is more important than ever for female yogis to share their empirical experiences as a basis for other women to understand and have faith in the benefits of the practice.

Let yourself be inspired by these mothers' stories, and know that what they achieved is within your reach. If you are a man, pass these stories on to the women in your life.

This book serves as a medium for these amazing women to share their stories. It is not a way to tell people what they should or should not do during their pregnancy. It is merely a way to share the stories of women who have had proven benefits of yoga. It is also important to note that none of the women that appear in this book started practicing yoga when they became pregnant. They had already been practicing, so their bodies adapted to the practice more easily as they maintained their healthy routines.

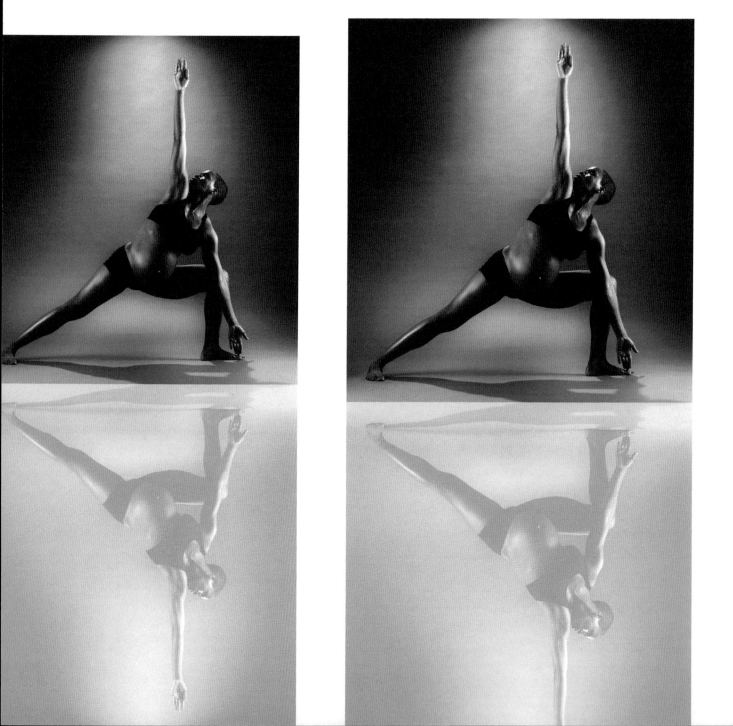

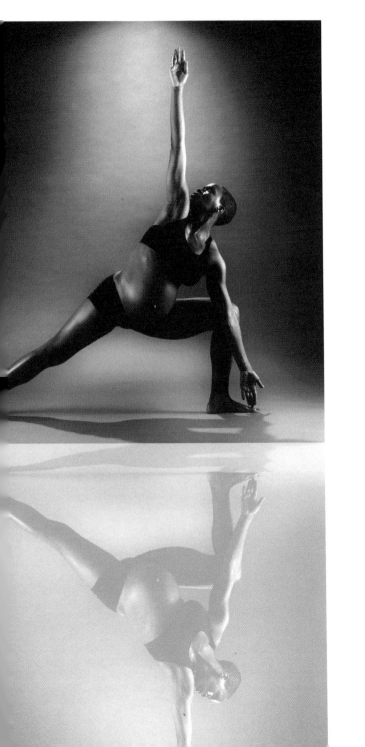
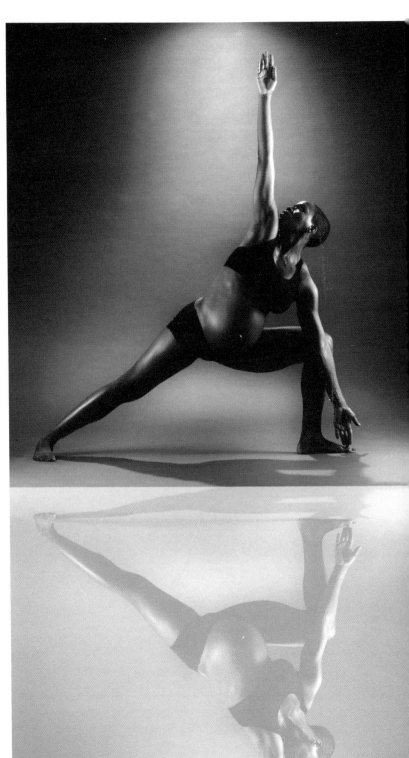

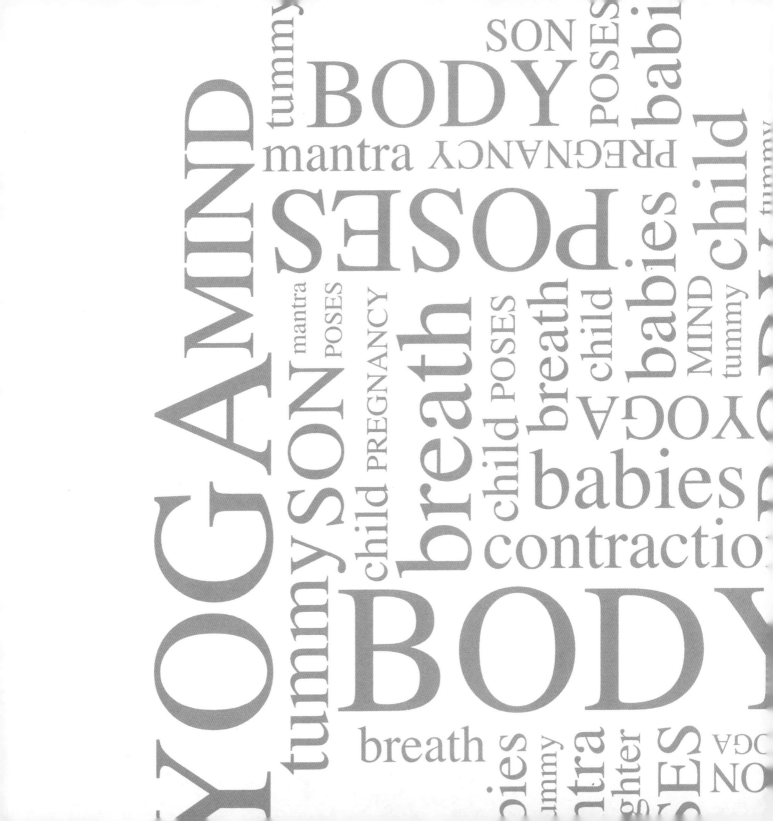

YOGA PREGNANCY

mantra breath babies
breath
babies contractions MIND
child breath
SON babies
contractions
daughter MIND
SON MIND POSES
mantra
contractions

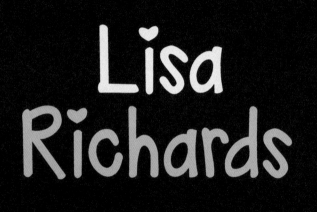

Lisa Richards

Yoga helped me give birth to two beautiful children; Sawyer and Stella.

The principles of yoga have helped me through a lot in my life. I see my yoga practice as the greatest analogy for living. It has helped me stay present and breathe during the most physically, emotionally, and spiritually challenging times. I used my yogic breathing and balance while approaching the summit of Mt. Kilimanjaro. I've been able to breathe, feel, and stay present during the passing of loved ones. But most significantly and memorably, yoga helped me give birth to two beautiful children: Sawyer and Stella.

For some women, pregnancy is beautiful with no complications. For others, it's challenging from beginning to end. Just like in yoga practice, you have your good days, and you have your off days. Many of the challenges you face during pregnancy can be equated with those that have been overcome in the yoga room. From the beginning, you deal with nausea (think holding camel pose for three minutes until you think you're going to puke), your body changes almost on a daily basis (think of the difference one day can make in your chair pose) and, of course, the hormones (feeling like you're going to lose it if you have to hold a hip-opening pose for a second longer). For me, the practice of yoga and the principles behind the practice were what I leaned on during both of my pregnancies.

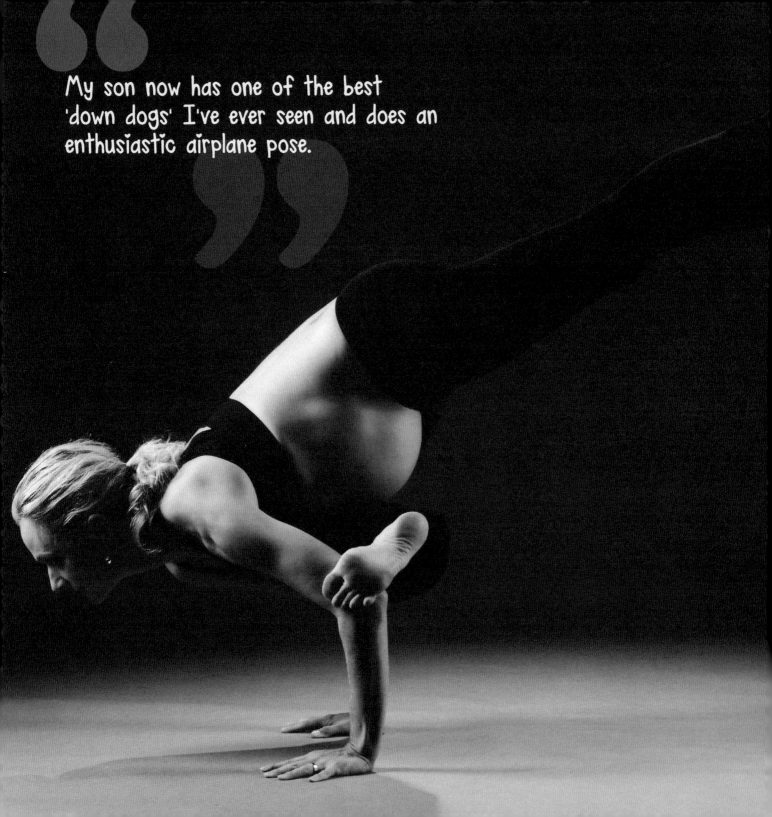

"My son now has one of the best 'down dogs' I've ever seen and does an enthusiastic airplane pose.

" I have never felt stronger or more intuitive than I did while pregnant. I think yoga empowered me to connect with the growing baby inside of me and embrace all of the (not so glamorous) changes with confidence and wonder. "

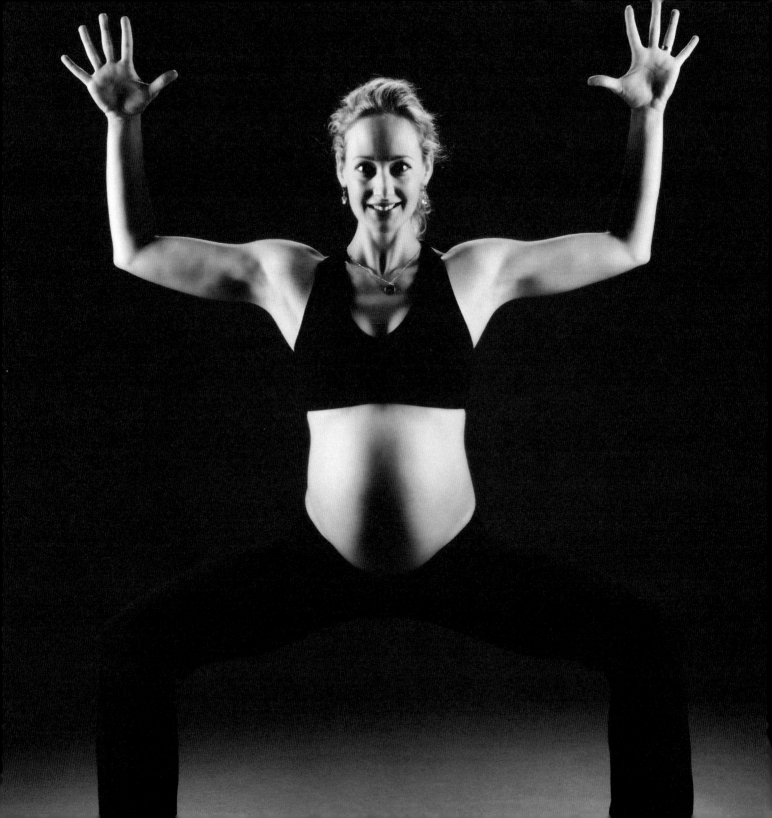

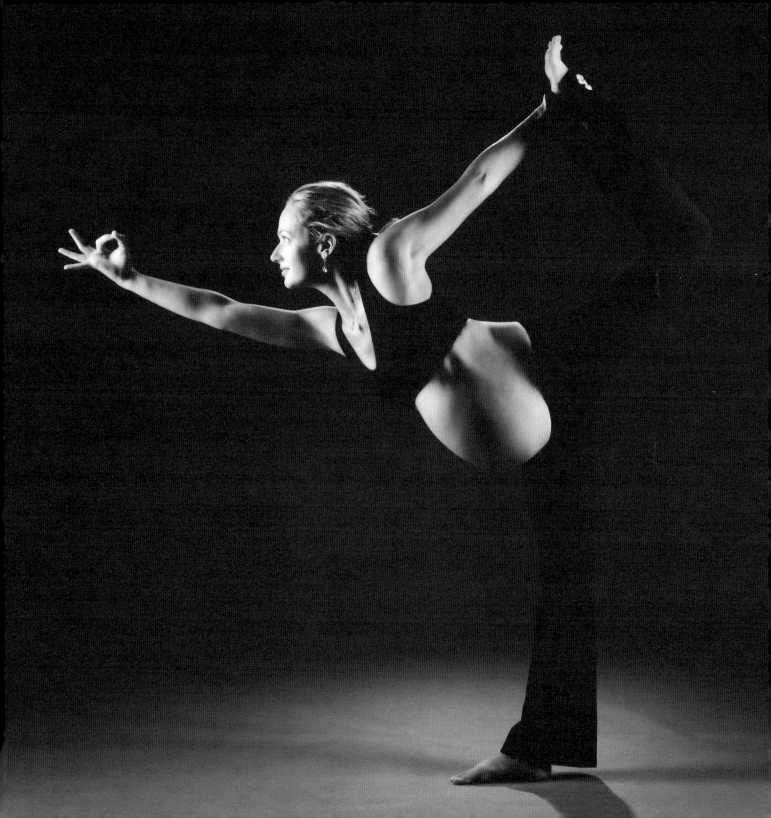

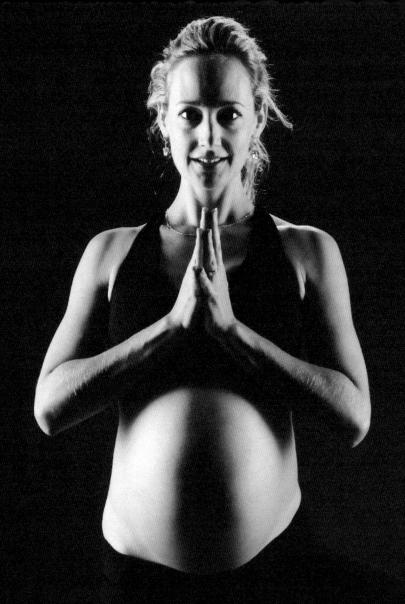

"I was back in the yoga room within weeks and practicing almost at the level I had before pregnancy."

When I became pregnant with my first child, I had been practicing yoga for 12 years and teaching for eight. What I love about yoga is the rhythmic sequence that allows you to find a place of meditation while in motion. There's a Rumi poem where one line states, "Don't push the river; it flows on its own." This is one tenant I tried to keep in mind while pregnant with both babies. By surrendering to the intuition and strength within my body and trying not to force anything, I was able to stay present and focused through my pregnancies.

During my pregnancies, my practice changed. Some postures, like a simple forward bend or extended side angle pose, needed modifying. Others were surprisingly easy. With the weight of my body growing and shifting, I found that I craved inversions like handstands and forearm stands. Taking a few moments upside down to resist gravity made a huge difference in how my shoulders and hips felt. I listened to my body and was gentle with it, but I was also not afraid to keep using it.

With my first pregnancy, I was able to continue most postures as I had pre-pregnancy, but I found that there was a lot of fear about pregnant women doing too much, or over-exerting themselves. When I was seven months pregnant with my son, I remember a student getting nervous and asking me to stop doing a forearm stand. While I believe women need to be cautious and listen to that intelligent internal voice, I also believe we are not given enough credit for our strength. I had never felt stronger or more intuitive than I did while pregnant. I think yoga empowered me to connect with the growing baby inside of me and embrace all of the (not so glamorous) changes with confidence and wonder.

Just as every yoga practice is different, so is every pregnancy. With my second pregnancy, I felt the need to modify more postures and slow down a bit more. I found hip-opening, supine, and prone postures, like pigeon, to be what I craved most. If I was going to flip upside down, I found I needed the wall to do so. Rather than judging the difference in my experiences, I felt lucky enough to embrace the voice that was telling me what was best for my body's needs.

I labored for 30 hours with my first child and 11 hours with my second. Besides my husband, my breath was my best partner. I did goddess pose against a wall during contractions, all the while useing my yogic breathing. My breath helped me to focus and be strong. The sound of it was almost like a mantra. I used my breath to stay present during all of my contractions as they became longer and more intense. In a way, I was able to become lost in my breath, and it carried me through even when I thought I wasn't going to be able to keep going.

At times, both birth experiences seemed like never-ending marathons. I am positive there is no way I would have been able to go 30 hours and 11 hours—without medical intervention—if I didn't have my yoga practice. Physically I was spent, but I kept finding reserves I never knew I possessed. Many times in class I have noticed that our minds give in way before our bodies do. If we tell ourselves we're tired or unable to keep going, the mind fools the body. But if we can turn off the mind and tap into our body, our potential is unbelievable. I remember finishing an intense contraction and feeling surprised that I had made it through, and then I felt empowered as I waited for the next one. Eventually, the apprehension of labor wore off, and I was able to approach it with a warrior spirit. I remember the moment both of my children were born so vividly. It was the biggest release of joy, fatigue, elation, amazement—a euphoric exhale.

I credit my yoga practice for quick healing after the birth. I was back in the yoga room within weeks and practicing almost at the level I had before pregnancy. My son now has one of the best down dogs I've ever seen and does an enthusiastic airplane pose. Once my daughter is able, I'm sure she will be doing her yoga poses early as well.

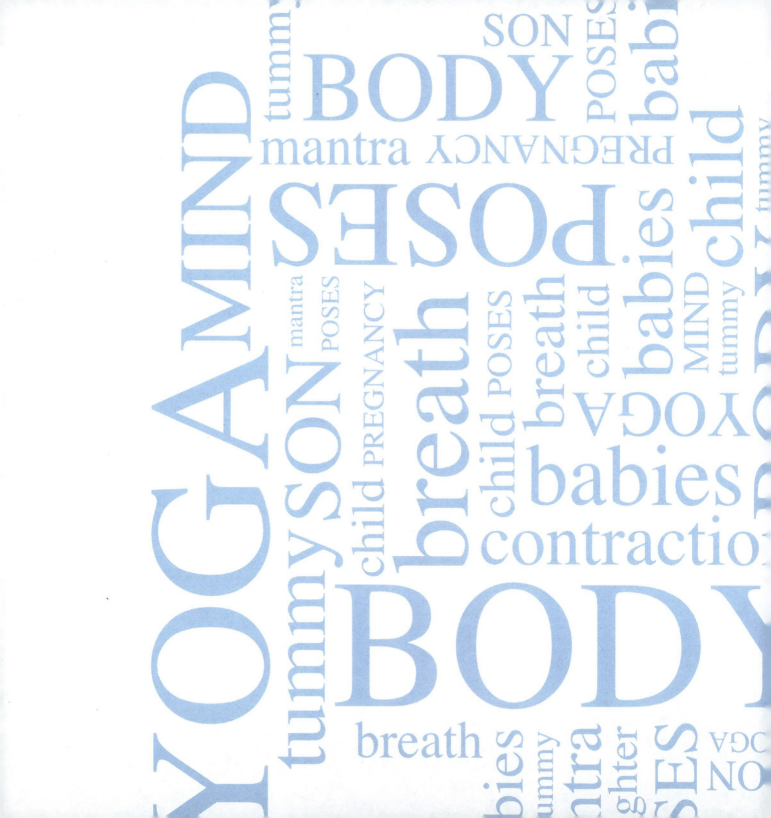

mantra breath babies contractions breath YOGA breath PREGNANCY SON babies mummy child babies contractions MIND contractions daughter MIND SON MIND POSES contractions mantra breath

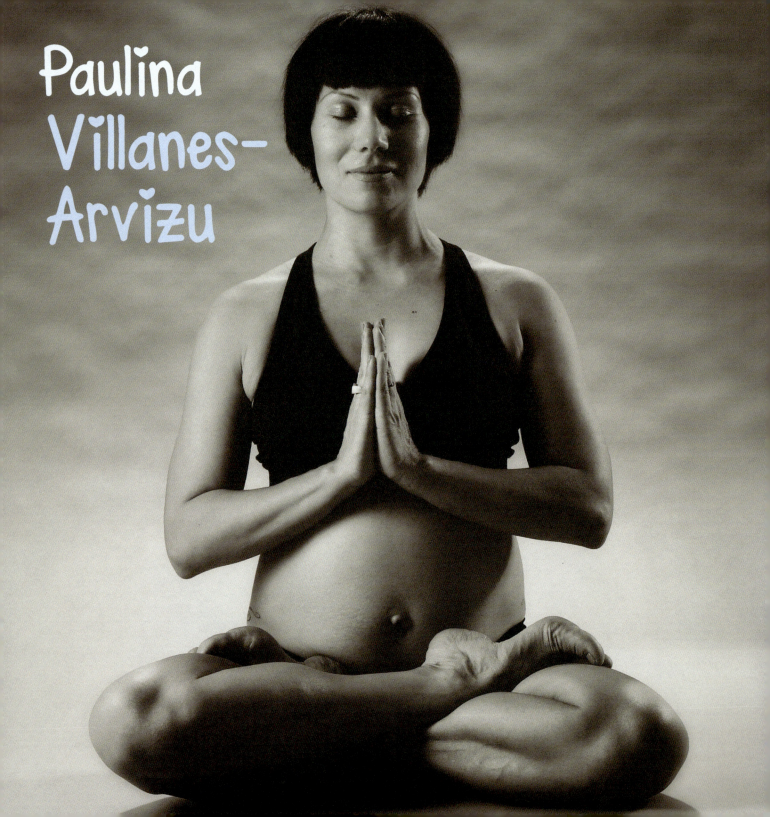

It is a pleasure to share the experiences of my three pregnancies. I only practiced yoga while I was pregnant with Rey and of course had a completely different experience than with my first two children.

My first two pregnancies were not easy, especially in comparison to the third. Psychologically, they were completely exhausting. For the entire nine months of pregnancy and six months after giving birth, my hormones changed abruptly from one state to another. My temper was intolerable; I did not know how to control myself. I remember asking myself, "Why do I feel angry?" but I could never find a reason for it. My pregnancy was technically "healthy," but I had no control over my emotions and couldn't bring myself to a state of mind that would be beneficial for the baby.

Walking was difficult during my first two pregnancies, even during the early stages. I felt a very strong pain in my lower back, so I walked as little as possible. I also developed a calcium deficiency in the hip area that required painkillers and the possibility of surgery. My doctor told me that, physiologically, my body was not designed to bear another child, and that a third pregnancy could cause serious health problems. I didn't like how this sounded and made a firm decision to try to find an alternative cure.

This is how I found and fell in love with yoga. From the very first class, I was hooked. Two years into my yoga practice, my body was in balance and apparently ready for a new pregnancy. It was during this time that I found out a new baby was on its way. My third experience was wonderful. I was happy every day, and I could literally feel the development of the baby in my belly. I felt an unexplainable connection to the baby and a deep appreciation for the presence. Practicing yoga daily made me understand how strong my body was and that it could sustain the development of a new being. The 90-minute Bikram practice filled me with the energy I needed for the everyday activities with my children. When I found out I was pregnant, I kept practicing but stopped pressing in or contracting my abdomen and stomach. I wanted to keep doing my practice, but I realized that some parts of it would have to change.

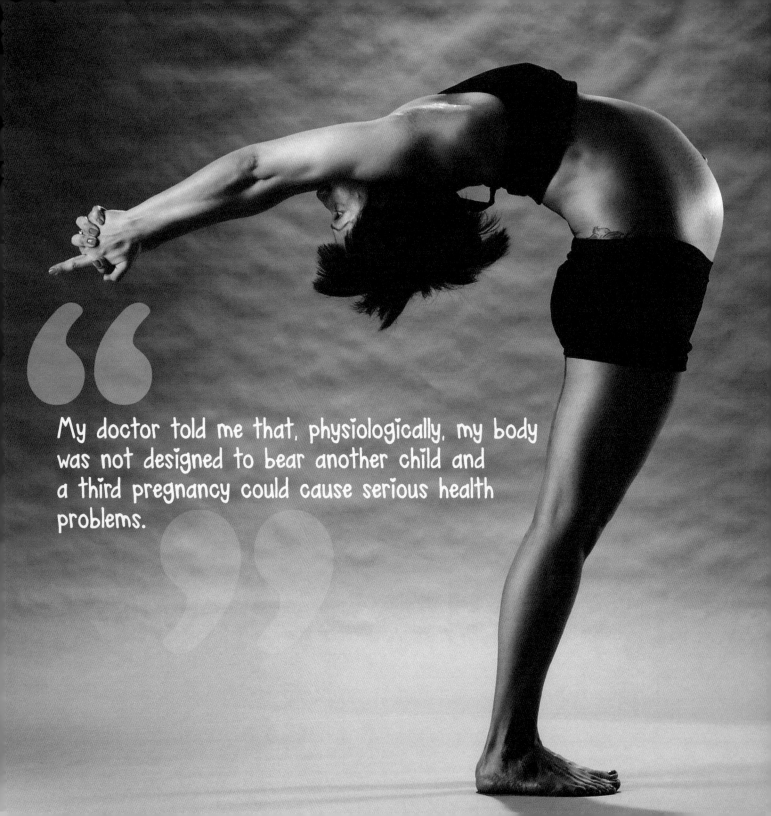

> Practicing yoga daily made me understand how strong my body was and that it could sustain the development of a new being. The 90 minute practice filled me with the energy I needed for the every day activities with my children.

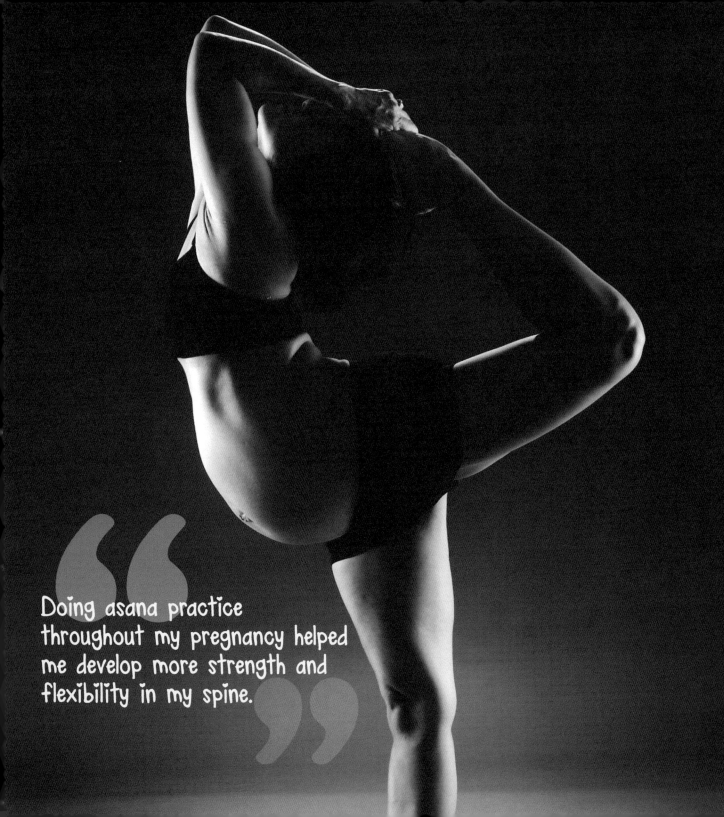

"Doing asana practice throughout my pregnancy helped me develop more strength and flexibility in my spine."

While the baby developed in my belly, I consciously kept altering the positions to what my body and the baby wisely required. The moment I felt pressure in my abdomen, I would give space for a little stretching of the body so the baby would have oxygen circulation and enough room to keep moving. Although each yoga posture only lasted for a few seconds I would listen carefully to my body and come out of the posture when I felt I had reached my limit for the day. On the day of labor, I felt a special energy between the baby and me. I started the day teaching a 7 a.m. yoga class. At 9 a.m., I took a class and was amazed by my flexibility. Postures that had been impossible during my entire pregnancy seemed easy. At 1 p.m., I went to a friend's baby shower, and at 4 p.m. I fixed a stroller for my children. At 7 p.m., my water broke, and at 11:01 p.m., my new baby Rey was born. It was a day full of a special energy which I would love to feel again in the future. A long and beautiful day!

Doing asana practice throughout my pregnancy helped me develop more strength and flexibility in my spine. Backbends, for example, became easier to perform because of the natural curve that forms when the baby's weight is the front area of the lower spine. Even now that pregnancy is over, I still keep that flexibility, and it helps heal the calcium deficit in my hips.

After Rey was born, the doctor told me I could go back to practicing my yoga class normally. I did not feel my body was ready to go back, so I waited almost two weeks to take my first class. I began practicing slowly—one class a week, and then two, and so on. My body told me to take it slow, and I respected what it needed.

After a pregnancy is over, your body is still in a process of transformation. In order for this transformation to happen, you need to listen to what your body wants. Be patient. Your body will go back to what it was before when you least expect it.

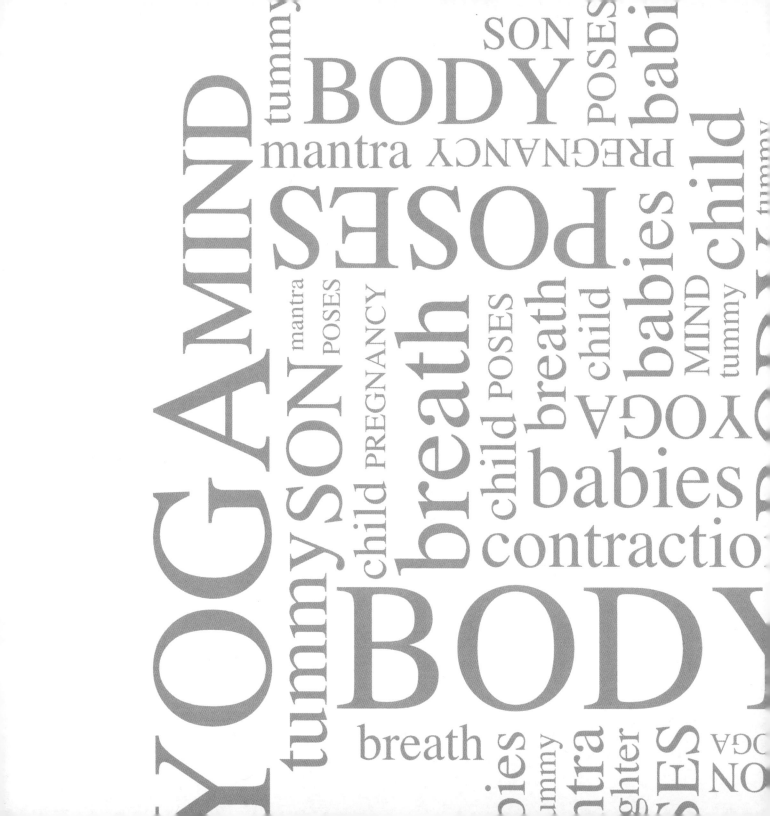

mantra babies contractions breath babies contractions MIND breath YOGA breath PREGNANCY SON babies child contractions daughter MIND jimmy SON MIND POSES mantra breath

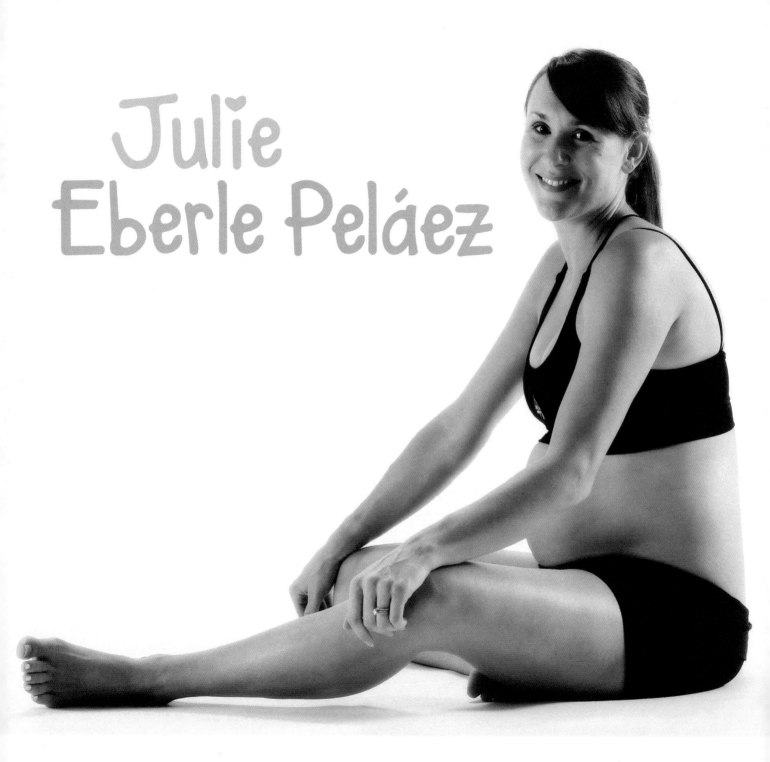

Everyone says childbirth and labor are like running a marathon. As my husband said, I just happened to run a very fast marathon. In many aspects, I feel blessed to have had a fast birth in our home nestled up against the Flatirons in beautiful Boulder, Colorado. We initially called our midwife at 9 a.m. She recommended breakfast and a walk among other things that we never got to, like going to the store, making up our birthing bed and space, and creating my birth altar. Having prepared mentally for my birth through the practice of yoga, I was able to stay lighthearted through my early labor, even laughing at some of the absurdities. At one point on our walk, we stopped when I had a particularly powerful contraction.

We had our dog, Chica, with us. The sun was shining. It was a glorious Friday. It just so happened we had stopped near a bus stop. So there I was, hunched over my husband, breathing deeply, the dog's leash wrapped around us, when the bus came to a stop. We had a good laugh at how this must have looked to the passengers. Around noon, we called our midwife again to let her know that things had progressed. Her advice was simply to figure out how to relax between contractions. My immediate thought was, "no problem; it's just like savasana."

It gave me time to envision my perfect birth. It gave me time to meditate on affirmations like, "my body knows exactly what to do," and, "I courageously surrender to the power of my body," and "I open to the energy and life force of birth." These affirmations carried me through active labor and delivery. I didn't focus on the intensity or the "pain-like sensation" (as we call it in yoga). I just stayed positive.

Years of practicing yoga and training my mind to choose positive thoughts prepared me for this. In yoga we learn to get into the zone, and was I ever in the zone during labor. It was completely surreal and amazing. I was so in "it" that when my midwife arrived she saw my body push. I guess they call these "expulsions." I wasn't forcing a push—my body was just doing it. It was amazing. It's like I completely surrendered and let my body do the work. Being able to have this state of mind is 1,000 percent because of my yoga practice.

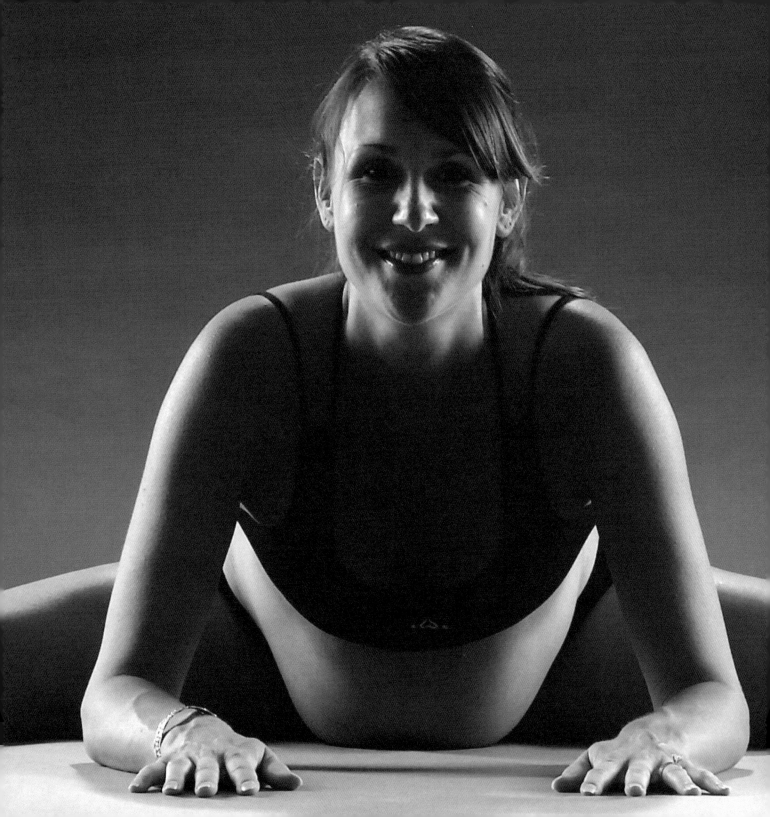

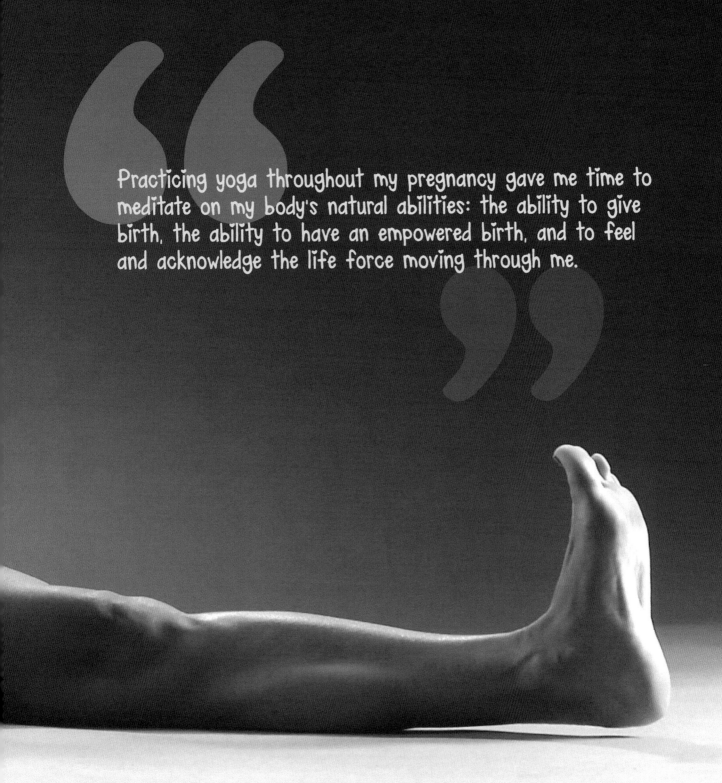

> Practicing yoga throughout my pregnancy gave me time to meditate on my body's natural abilities: the ability to give birth, the ability to have an empowered birth, and to feel and acknowledge the life force moving through me.

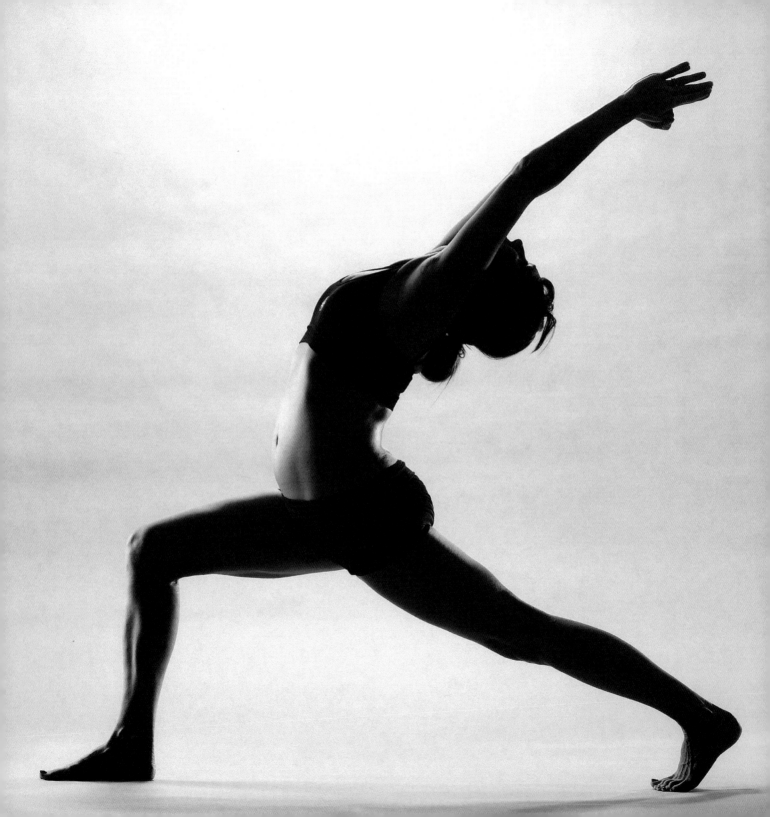

> I wasn't forcing a push, my body was just doing it. It was amazing. It's like I completely surrendered and let my body do the work. Being able to have this state of mind is 1,000 percent because of my yoga practice.

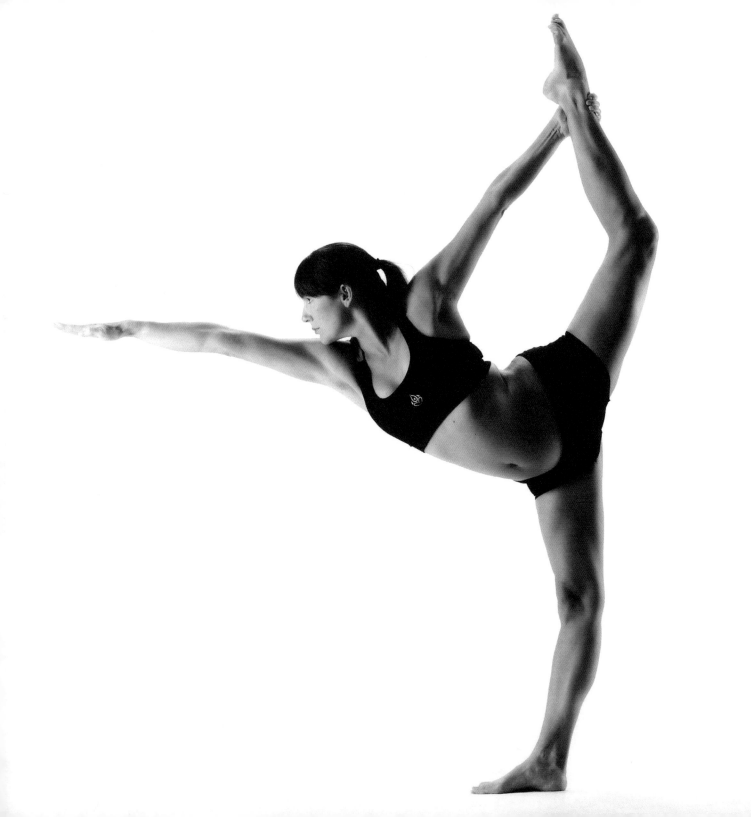

I can honestly say being pregnant was one of the most profound times in my life. It was because of my yoga practice that I had time to really appreciate my changing body. The time allowed me to meditate on my baby, my body, and my birth. I remember looking into the mirror during half moon pose. I thought I could see the outline of the baby when I stretched to the right side; I could see the curve of his body along the left side of my belly. I felt so much love for him. I had a mantra from early on that my midwife suggested: "head down, back to belly and hands at heart center." This was the most ideal position for birth, and I repeated it over and over and over again. I also spent much of the last few months of my pregnancy focusing on letting go. On allowing my hips to expand, letting go of the perineum muscles, letting everything hang down, and allowing gravity to do its part. When it came time for labor, this was now a natural thing for me to do, and ultimately I am sure this is what helped me move the baby down and out so quickly.

During yoga, I felt deeply connected to the baby and to the miracle of life itself. I felt great throughout my pregnancy without the typical complaints of high blood pressure, nausea, swelling, and constipation. Instead, I was able to focus on the miracle growing inside me. It was special to be in the yoga room looking at my changing, growing, abundant body. I felt so privileged to be growing a baby. It was during my yoga practice that I really got to connect to these feelings.

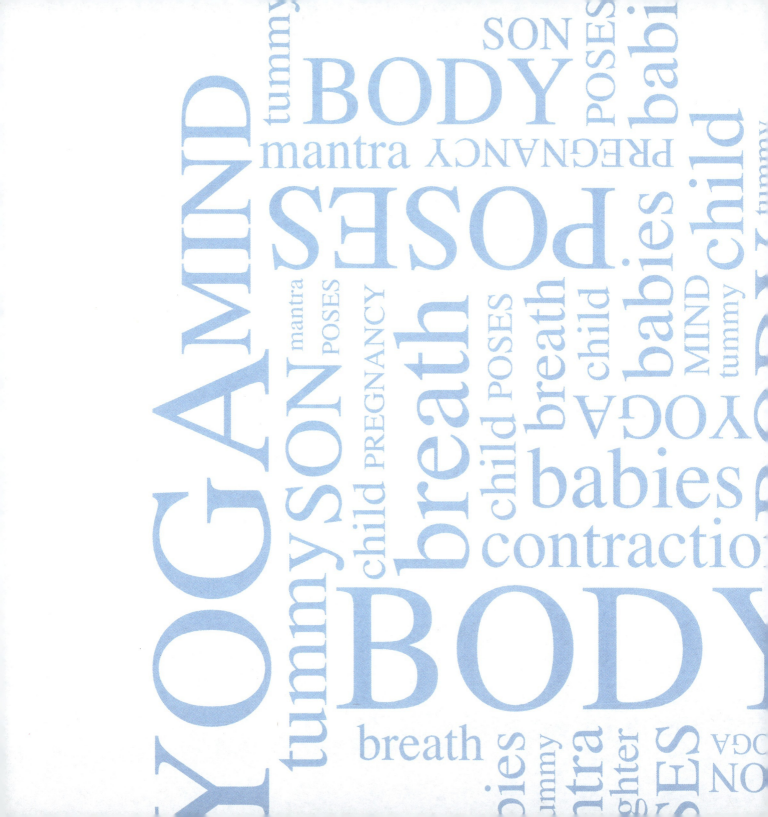

mantra breath babies contractions breath YOGA breath PREGNANCY SON babies
babies contractions MIND
child
SON MIND POSES
mantra
contractions daughter MIND
breath

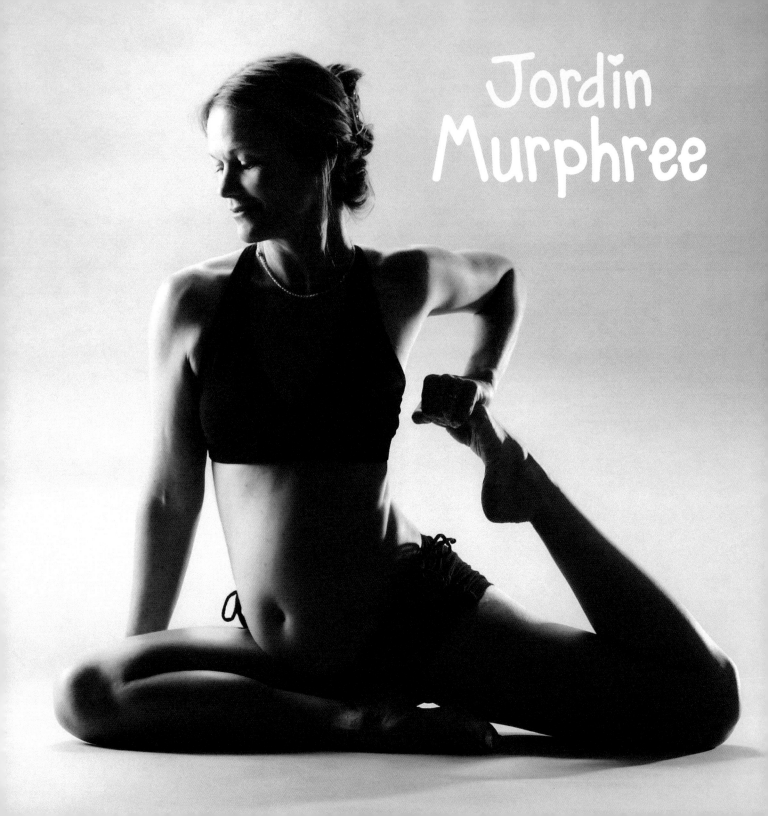

During my pregnancy, people at the yoga studio would always say, "Yoga is going to make your labor and delivery so much easier, don't you think?" I would answer, "I'm sure it will help me in some way." Of course, I hoped I was going to have this totally smooth, easy delivery because I practice yoga. But I also thought it was not necessarily within my control. Just because I do a lot of yoga did not guarantee that my birth would be a piece of cake. My doula told me many times, "the labor fairy comes along and gives you the labor that is right for you and your baby." So that is what I tried to focus on: Instead of being attached to a specific outcome, I tried to focus on trusting that the birth would unfold in a way that was right for me and my baby. It was a challenge to not be attached. I wanted the most straightforward birth, and I wanted to do it without drugs. The one thing that I could and did control was choosing not to use drugs.

Practicing yoga was a fabulous way to prepare mentally and physically for childbirth. Doing yoga asanas was a way for me to experience deep relaxation and remain physically strong during my pregnancy. I think that having a daily practice for those nine months, when my body was going through huge changes, helped me keep up with the changes. Yoga gives me a connection to my body and helps me notice when something feels right or when something is amiss.

Throughout my pregnancy, I subscribed to a weekly email newsletter about what to expect with your changing pregnant body, and a lot of the advice was not positive: expect back pain, swollen ankles, high blood pressure, water retention, and general discomfort. This was not my experience. Physically, I felt great up to the last days before delivery. I honestly didn't really feel that big or that my body was that different. It makes me laugh now when I look at pictures of myself pregnant and see that I was huge, but at the time, I felt pretty normal and mobile. I definitely attribute this to my yoga practice.

Having those 90 minutes of Bikram to nurture myself on a daily basis was a gift. It helped me stay connected and grounded in reality during a time that was very surreal. The thought that I could grow a human being inside me was (and still is) mind-blowing.

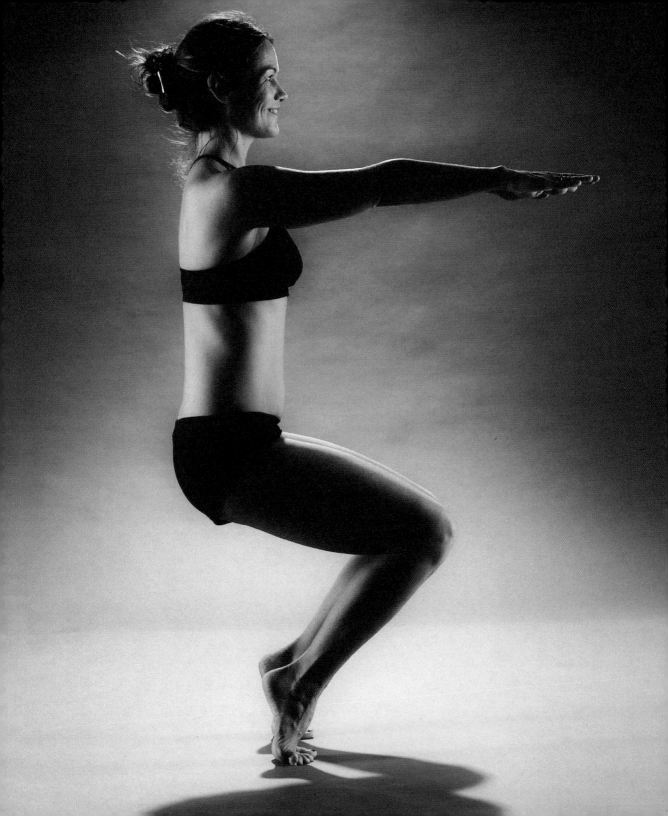

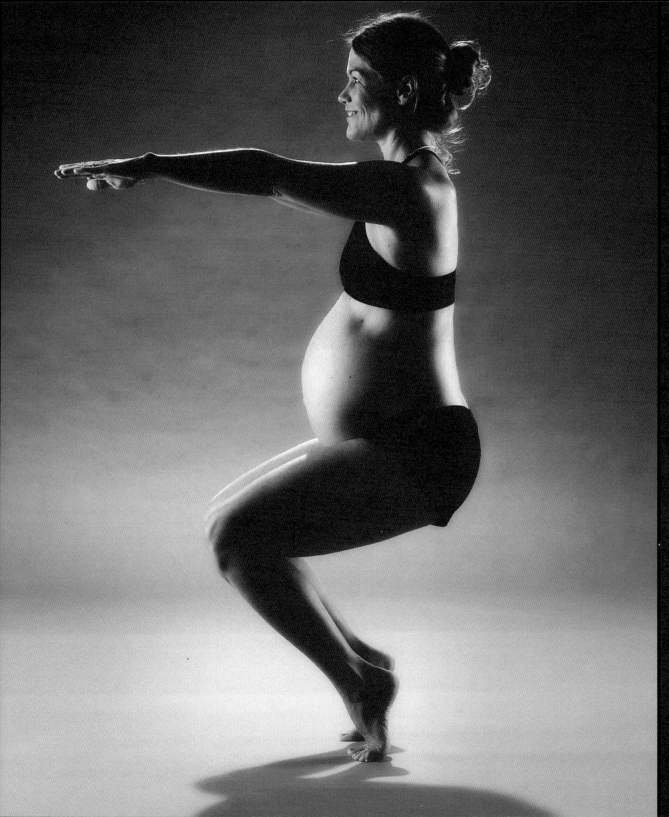

Seeing myself in the mirror every day and doing postures in a way that constantly reminded me there was a baby in there was a great way to help me connect with the baby. Often, during many of the savasanas, I could feel him moving, especially after camel and in the final savasana. That was a trip! I think he liked getting the flush of fresh blood and oxygen. I had the luxury of napping each day after class in final savasana for about 30 minutes. That time of being still and quiet was very refreshing and rejuvenating.

Physically, my yoga practice prepared me for what turned out to be a very active and "athletic" labor. Cassin, my baby, was in the occiput posterior position, which means the back of his head was towards my spine. Most babies in this position will turn over eventually, but for some reason he was already too far down in my pelvis and could not turn. This requires a few more centimeters of room than usual for the baby to make its way through the pelvis and down the birth canal. Babies facing the optimal direction can tuck their chin so just the crown of their head moves through. When in the posterior position, it is not possible for them to tuck their chin, so the oblong circumference of the head needs to move through. What this means for mama is a prolonged and more intense period of pushing, along with severe tearing of the perineal tissues. It is also extremely common for a baby in this position to be delivered via C-section.

I was determined to push my baby out rather than have surgery. I told the OB that I knew I could do it, and he agreed to let me try. He was very nervous, but he saw my determination and gave me the benefit of the doubt. I was able to do it after a whole day of what felt like running four marathons back to back without stopping. I had to stay in an upright squatting position for most of the labor, and push in order to bring Cassin down far enough. Gravity was my ally. I am so grateful I chose not to have drugs because with an epidural, you have no feeling in your legs and cannot use them. An epidural and a baby in the posterior position is a recipe for a C-section in most cases. It was years of practicing yoga that allowed me to be in a squatting position for a prolonged period of time and enabled me to eventually push Cassin out. Not only do I believe the yoga completely prepared me physically for giving birth, but, maybe more important, it gave me the mind strength and determination to get the job done. All those years of practicing to discipline my mind paid off in full force during my delivery. Anyone who has done the spine strengthening series in a hot yoga class knows that, at least at first, you absolutely dread each one.

You mull it over in your mind before the posture starts, think about how hard it is while you are doing it, and then decide that it is too hard and come out early. That was me the first year of my practice. Then, little by little, I noticed how much my mind played a role. I could choose to suffer through it, or turn my mind off and just do it. It felt so much better to do the latter. I found a direct correlation to that during my labor. Each contraction was like the longest, most challenging locus pose I've ever done, but about 100 times more intense. But I was not thinking about how much it hurt; I was just doing it. The time between the contractions was like the deepest, sweetest, most relaxing savasana ever experienced.

I remember saying to my husband and the doula how good I felt during the time between contractions. It was like I was floating on a cloud. I remember it being easy for me to be in the moment with the relaxation, not anticipating the next contraction. If I had not done that, there is no way I would have lasted through two and a half hours of pushing.

My physical strength and mental determination showed up for me in full force that day. The birth showed me I was capable of more than I ever knew. I certainly credit my years of yoga practice to that. Yoga philosophy speaks of the five aspects of the mind: faith, determination, concentration, self-discipline and willpower. Throughout the years, I've used those qualities to develop a nice standing head to knee and standing bow postures. But, so what, really? What is much more important, I believe, is that the things we practice and learn in the yoga room are true training for the bigger tasks in life.

One thing I enjoyed about practicing yoga asanas during my pregnancy was the creativity. While practicing in a class with other students, I modified each posture for carrying a baby. There are a few basic guidelines that all pregnant women should follow, but it is up to the individual to do what feels right at any given time. The pregnancy modifications are not a one-size-fits-all, and they change as the pregnancy progresses. For some, it would be appropriate to do certain things that would not be appropriate for others. For example, my friend ChauKei could go into wheel and stand up from wheel, in place of floor bow, all the way up to the ninth month. She has an unusually flexible and strong spine. I did wheel until the third trimester when it started to feel like it was too much.

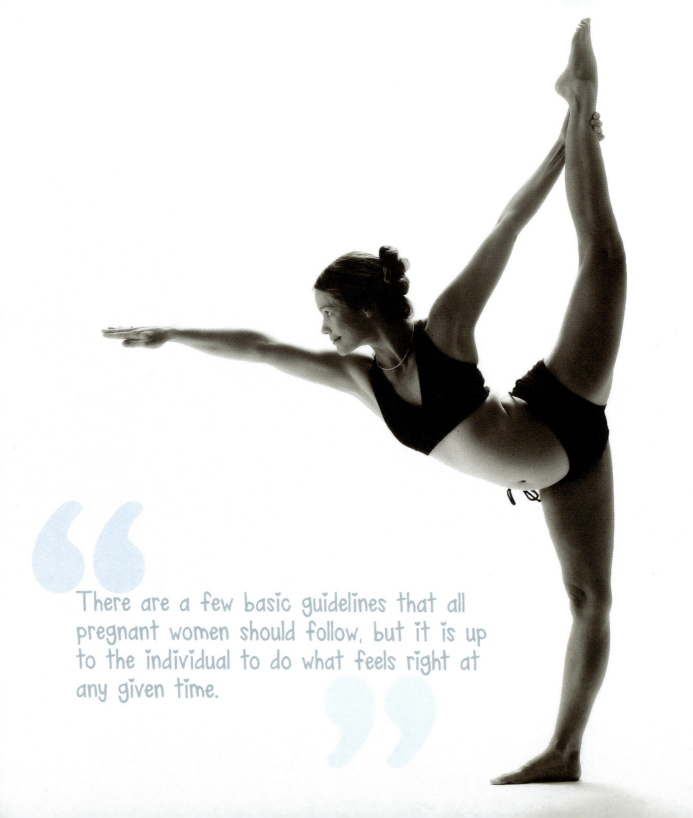

"There are a few basic guidelines that all pregnant women should follow, but it is up to the individual to do what feels right at any given time."

There are a few basic guidelines I suggest following when doing the pregnancy series. Do not suck in your stomach or use your abs too much. In the last trimester, especially, it is very important to "let the baby hang" so the baby can follow gravity as it gets closer to delivery. You do not want to create compression on the baby or restrict the flow of blood and oxygen. So, for example, toward the middle of the second trimester, postures like rabbit are no longer doable (for most women).

Be aware of your body temperature and don't overheat. The issue of body temperature is very controversial. Some think it is preposterous to practice yoga in a hot room. And it may not be appropriate for everyone. If you are new to the practice, starting a hot yoga style when you are pregnant is not ideal. But if you have had a regular practice before getting pregnant, for many it is totally fine. It's been proven that core body temperature does not necessarily rise during the class, and that's what pregnant women should be concerned about.

Because we sweat, the body can self regulate its core temperature. It would be different if you were in a hot tub where your body cannot release the heat. If there is a time when you do feel overheated, just leave the room. I think I did a time or two over the course of my pregnancy. This is not the time to push yourself in your practice. This is the time to relax and enjoy your changing body.

Practicing yoga throughout my pregnancy made the experience of being pregnant even more enjoyable. I am so grateful I was able to do it consistently, all the way up to the day before I delivered. I felt so good, and it helped me to keep in tune with my body. I wish all pregnant women could experience it.

Now that I have had my baby, I make it to yoga class twice a week. This is a huge change for me because for eight years, I was in there about five times a week. My asanas do not look or feel like they used to, but for now, I am not too concerned with that. I don't have childcare every day, and my priorities have shifted. Cassin is only going to be this young for a short period of time, and he is sweeter and more precious than I could have ever known. The love I feel for him is something I did not know existed. I feel at peace in my mind and in my heart. I know the hours of yoga that I practiced over the years helped to bring that as a focal point in my life, and that is here to stay.

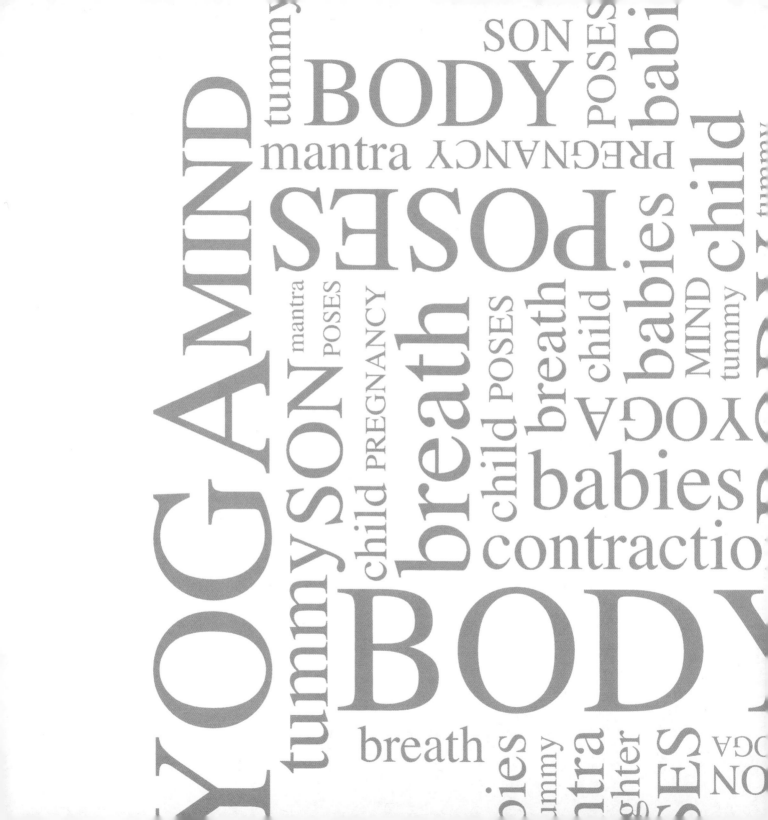

mantra breath babies contractions breath MIND YOGA breath PREGNANCY SON babies contractions babies contractions mantra child MIND daughter MIND mummy SON MIND POSES mantra breath

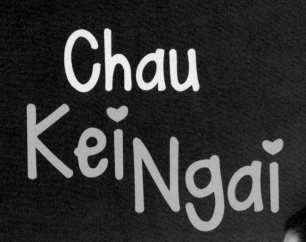

Chau Kei Ngai

> "Within my yoga practice I have overcome numerous challenges and I've watched myself transform and become capable of feats I didn't think I was capable of."

In June 2008, we found out I was one month pregnant. The same day, I did a yoga demonstration. I didn't know what was really going on in my body. All I knew was there was a pebble-like "being" inside my belly, and parallel with that I had total faith that I could keep practicing my yoga; I could not stop—not just then.

The next thing I did was buy the best-selling pregnancy book, "What to Expect When You're Expecting." It had good information; however, in the exercise section, it specifically said, "No hot yoga because of internal body temperature rises." But hot yoga is what I practice. At the time, I had been teaching for two years and practicing for four. I knew that our body temperature rises less than one degree because of the constant sweating. A normal person's body temperature can vary one degree throughout the day, depending on how active he or she is. So the advice given in that book made no sense to me, and it didn't stop me from doing my yoga.

I consider myself a yoga athlete. Sometimes I spend four or five hours a day in the yoga room, which exceeds the interest level for most modern yogis with busy lives. Within my yoga practice, I have overcome numerous challenges and watched myself transform and become capable of feats I didn't think I was capable of. This is true physical and emotional. Physically, I have found myself sturdy in postures I thought were beyond me. Emotionally, I found that I can breathe calmly through struggles, like I do in yoga class.

I also gained confidence in myself and who I am from my yoga practice. I took this confidence into my pregnancy. At first, I had very little knowledge about pregnancy and my own anatomy. A couple months into it, I actually asked a friend, "Where does the baby come out? From the front or the back?" I understood that there was a magnificent human being in my body, but beyond that I knew very little about how our bodies fit together and what I was in for. But I knew was that for nine months, he was a part of me, and I was capable of overcoming challenges.

I grew up in Hong Kong, China, until I was 15 years old. Hong Kong is a very modern city, and interestingly enough, even though we were brought up in Eastern culture, Western medicine was commonly practiced. Women go to the hospital for childbirth, and a great number of them have Cesarean sections, like in the West. When I told my family I planned to have a natural home birth, they were anxious about it.

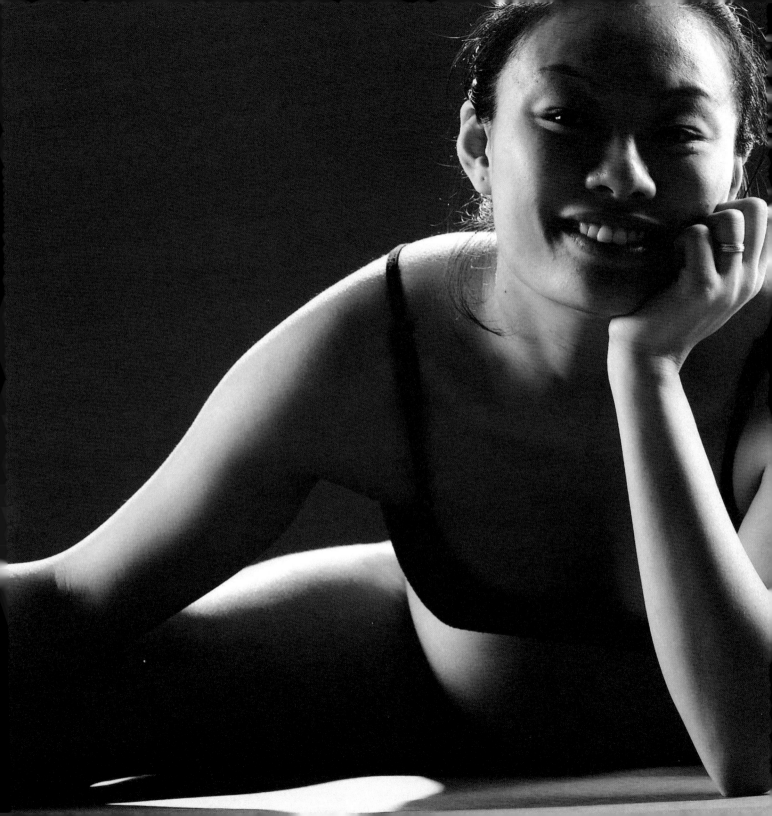

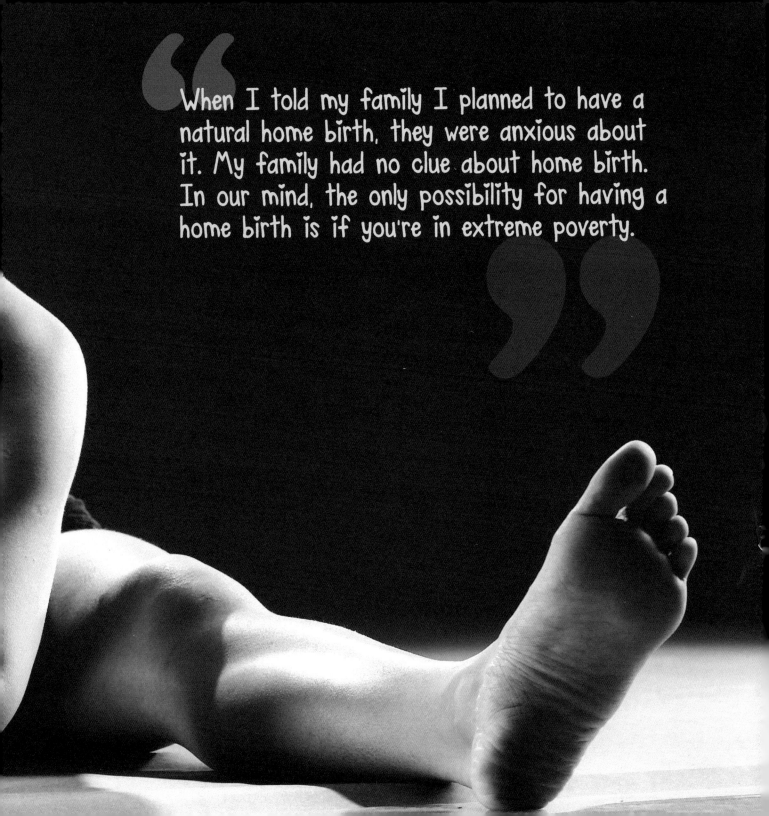

> "When I told my family I planned to have a natural home birth, they were anxious about it. My family had no clue about home birth. In our mind, the only possibility for having a home birth is if you're in extreme poverty."

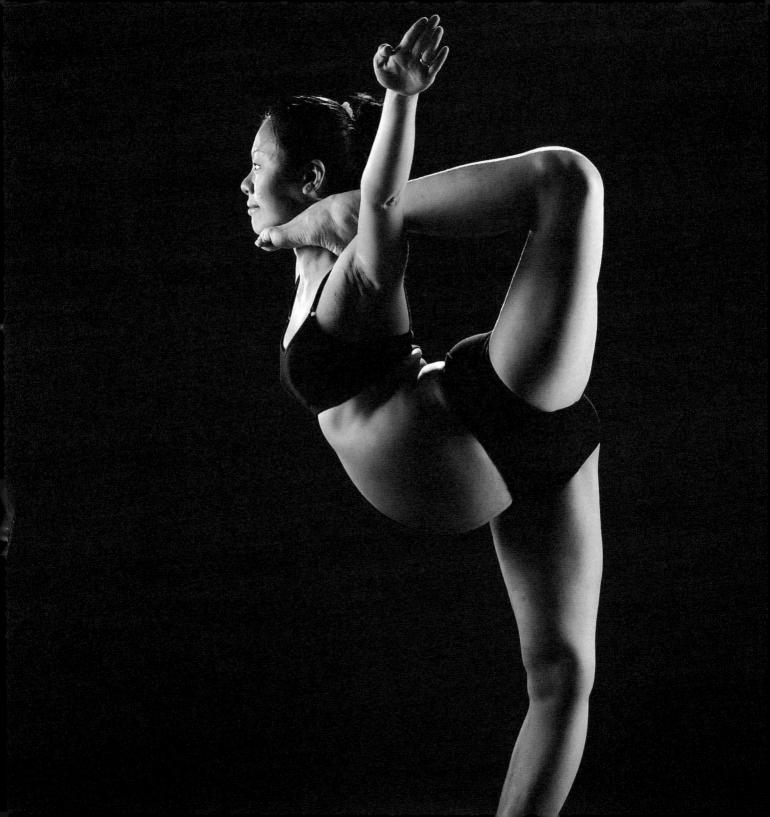

My family had no clue about home birth. In their mind, the only reason for having a home birth is if you're in extreme poverty. Their mentality was that only less fortunate people did not go to the hopital, and that denying the hospital was not a choice, but rather something people were forced into. During the years I spent practicing yoga in the West, I made friendships that turned my belief about hospitals upside down. The understanding of my own body and the nature of all beings was growing. Besides helping my strength, flexibility, and breathing technique, more important was the trust of the true inner strength, the core of my being. I knew I was going to do this without resistance and fear. I was so ready for this beautiful human experience and excited to share it with my family and friends.

In the yoga room during the pregnancy, I always thought that it was such a blessing that I was actually able to move my body the way I could. I practiced my yoga gently. In fact, if you ask my friends, they might not say so, because I was doing lots of advanced yoga postures; however, I was doing them with full awareness without pushing it, so I was gentle with myself.

A few months into the pregnancy, I found an amazing midwife named Yeni. Every time I left the appointment with her, I felt that I was doing the right thing for my baby. I had never feel healthier! Near the end of the pregnancy, Yeni encouraged me to gain more weight. I had already gained about 25 pounds, but Yeni said usually women usually gain 30 pounds or more. I knew I had gained a healthy amount of weight because I was still doing yoga, and I'm also naturally petite. I knew that from practicing hot yoga, I burn more calories than a normal woman. I felt strong! At that point, I didn't have any swollen feet or ankles or insomnia, and I only had minimal backaches with my giant belly. I just felt great throughout the entire pregnancy.

On January 18, 2009, I did a pregnant yoga demonstration. A while later, at 3 a.m. on January 19, my water broke. Twenty-four hours later, my first contraction started. Another 24 hours later, Osiris was born in the water of our bathtub at home. The labor was seamless, and the contractions were like waves coming and going. I related it to yoga class: asana and savasana. I learned how to let go in yoga. Osiris was born in perfect health. He was bright and happy. After Osiris was born, I continued practicing. If I had stopped practicing yoga, my body would not have bounced back so quickly. Today, I'm in perfect health, and Osiris is a magnificent human being, as we expected.

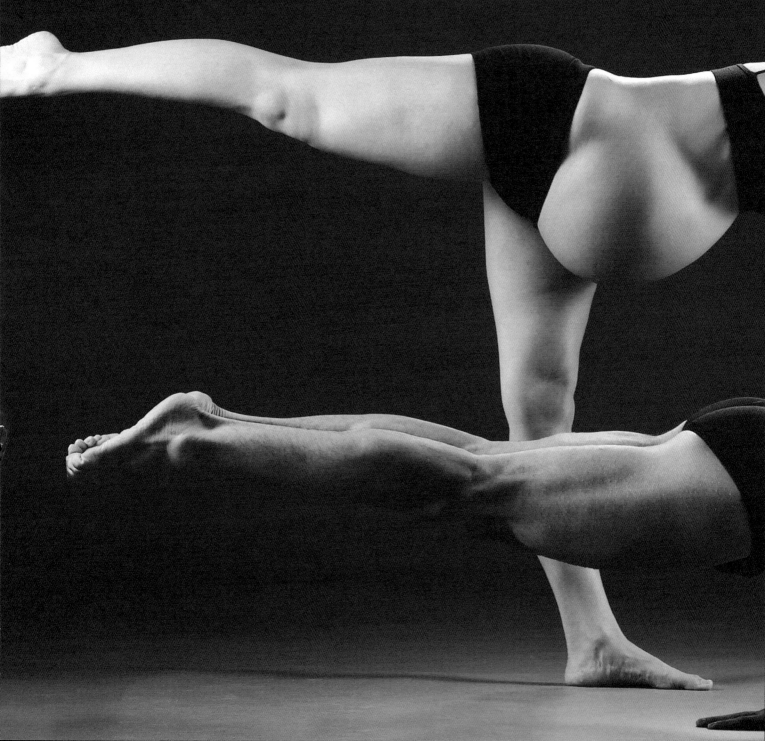

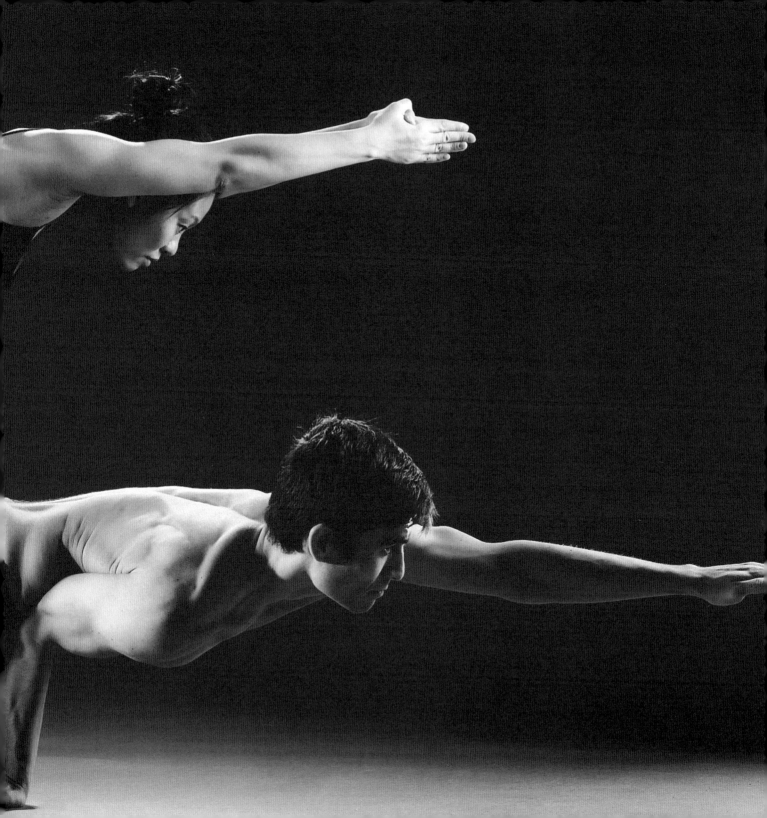

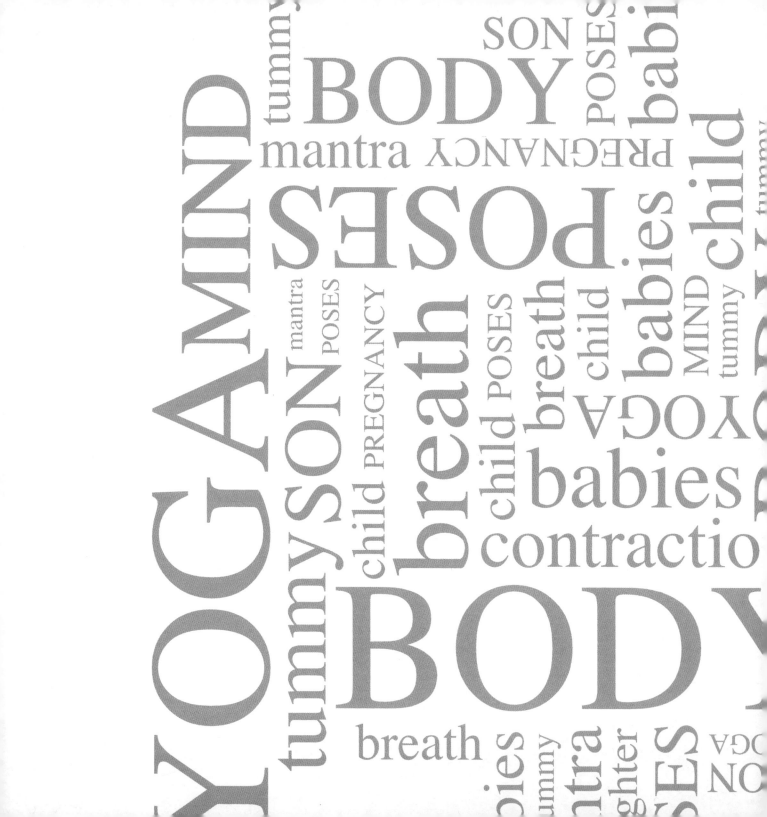

YOGA PREGNANCY

babies breath contractions mantra child MIND SON POSES daughter mantra

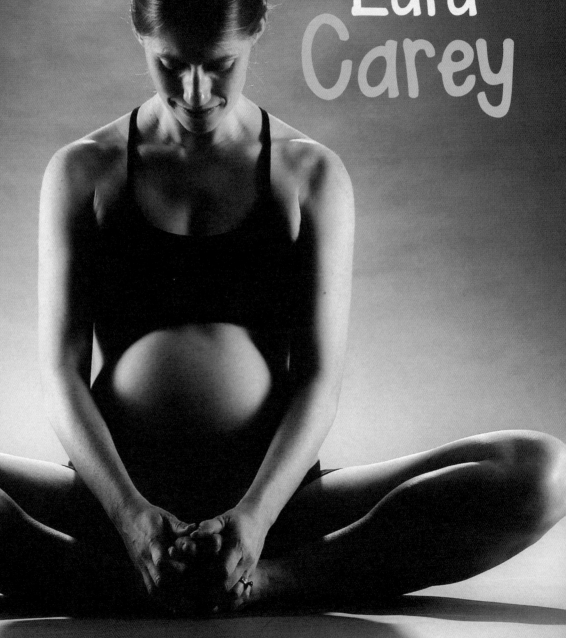
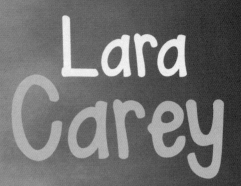

Yoga found me eight years ago. I was an East Coaster and had just moved to Boulder. Eager to meet new friends, I accepted an invitation from a friend to join her for a yoga class. Wow! I hated it. I had never done yoga before. It felt so awkward, and I was very uncomfortable in my own skin. The class was especially challenging because it consisted of practicing yoga while standing in front of a mirror for 90 minutes, sweaty and red-faced. Somehow, I made it through the first class, but I vowed not to do it again—ever. Yet, I still found myself nodding my head in agreement to my second invitation to next week's class.

I went one to three times a week for several years; it became a part of my life. I loved the way I felt after class. Getting to class was always the hardest part. The energy of the other people in class always got me through, no matter how tough of a time I was having. After a while, I actually felt good during class, not just after the class had ended.

About four years ago, I started taking classes more frequently, generally every other day. Sometimes I'd go on stints of practicing every day. And sometimes I'd practice twice a day. Sometimes I'd miss weeks at a time. But my practice has been fairly steady over the last four years. I certainly never had the foresight to realize how much impact my practice would have on my pregnancy and birth. If I'd had the foresight, I might have started practicing yoga for those reasons alone. Like most women who become pregnant, I started reading. I picked up several pregnancy books, one of which was "What to Expect When You're Expecting." It specifically said to avoid hot yoga. I was surprised because three expecting women were in the hot room where I practice. One had recently given birth to a healthy boy. They all looked so much healthier and more comfortable than the average pregnant woman, so I decided not to follow the advice I had read.

At first, I wondered if I might not be able to practice the whole way through my pregnancy. All the pregnant women I'd seen practicing were teachers, and I was a mere student. I finally decided I would go until it didn't feel right. For me, my last pregnant class turned out to be on a Thursday afternoon, and I went into labor a day and a half later on Saturday morning. Our amazing little son, Ethan, was born Saturday night.

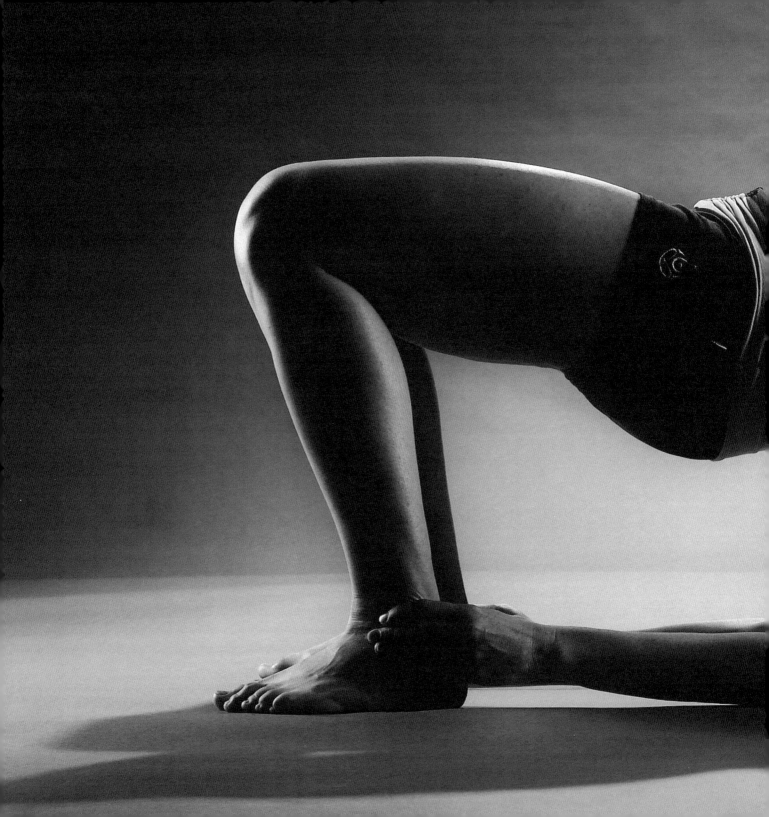

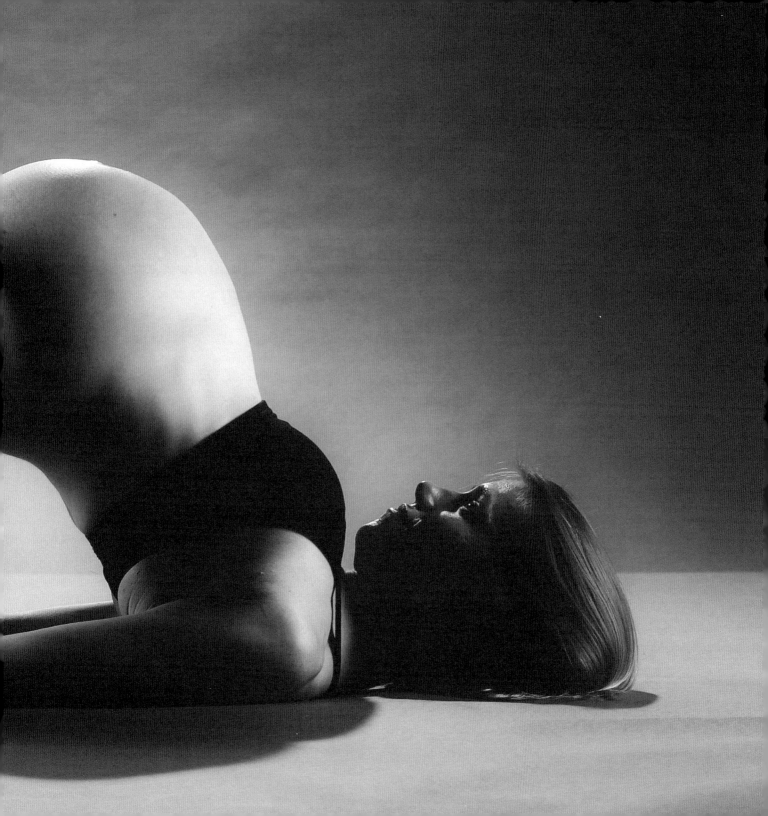

One skill you practice during every minute of yoga class is how to stay with your breath. Using your breath, you can master the discomfort of the heat, deepen stretches, and find your focus. You connect with your body. During the final stage of labor, the pushing phase, I heavily relied on my ability to stay with my breath. Ethan weighed eight and a half pounds when he was born—not a small baby. Breathing with the contractions allowed them to work just as evolution intended. This phase of labor was intense for me, but I had a sense of calm inside. As soon as Ethan was born, the physical intensity switched off, and I was "in the calm" with my gorgeous son lying on my chest.

Birth gave me such enormous respect for my body, for the amazing task it had undergone and how beautifully and perfectly it had performed. A regular practice keeps the machine doing exactly what it is intended to do. My yoga practice kept my body tuned perfectly throughout my pregnancy, and I birthed a healthy, thriving boy. The human body is incredible, especially the female body when it comes to reproduction. Practicing yoga kept my body tuned up and kept me in tune with my body. I was amazed by my body's recovery. The muscle memory snapped my body back into shape. I must note that I rested for a good while. For the first two weeks, I did not get out of bed except to go to the bathroom. It was five weeks after birth when I returned to yoga class. By 10 weeks post-birth, I was only five pounds more than my pre-pregnancy weight. Weight is not, of course, always the best measure, especially considering how the body changes post-birth. But I do attribute the ease in getting back in shape to a steady yoga practice. I am grateful because feeling healthy and strong is a huge benefit when you take care of a little one all day, every day. Being pregnant while doing yoga turned out to have more benefits than just physical ones. It turned out to be an incredible way to deepen my practice.

My first trimester was the most uncomfortable. I found that "morning sickness" was a misnomer; for me, it was a nauseous feeling all day. But I kept going to yoga. Sometimes it meant sitting out several postures. And sometimes it meant leaving the room and nibbling on some pretzels in the locker room. I had to listen very closely to my body. Throughout class, I would ask myself repeatedly, "What is my body trying to tell me?" I found that being pregnant allowed me to truly honor what my body was telling me.

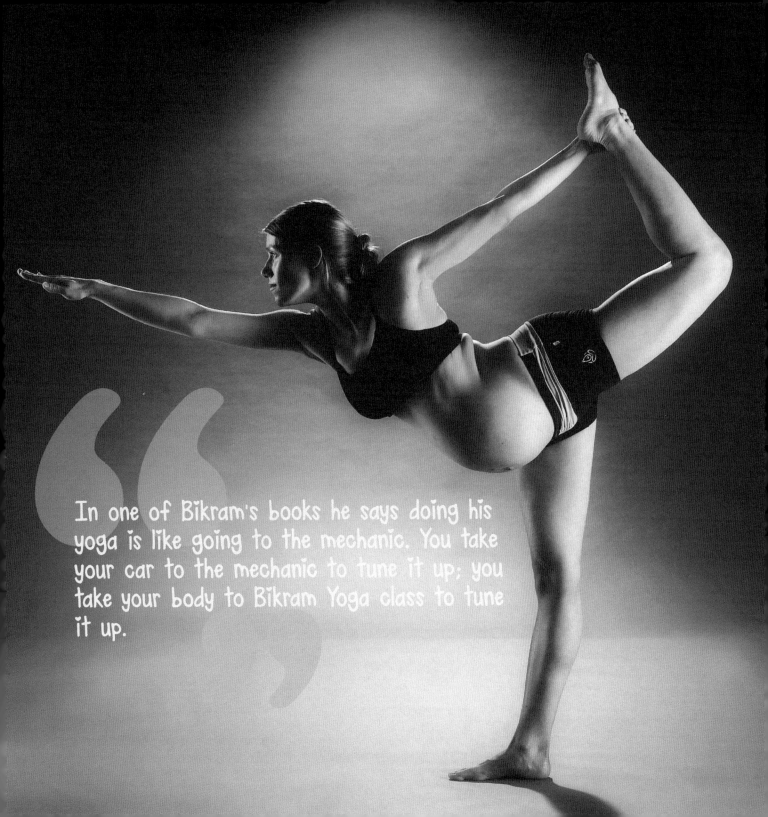

"In one of Bikram's books he says doing his yoga is like going to the mechanic. You take your car to the mechanic to tune it up; you take your body to Bikram Yoga class to tune it up."

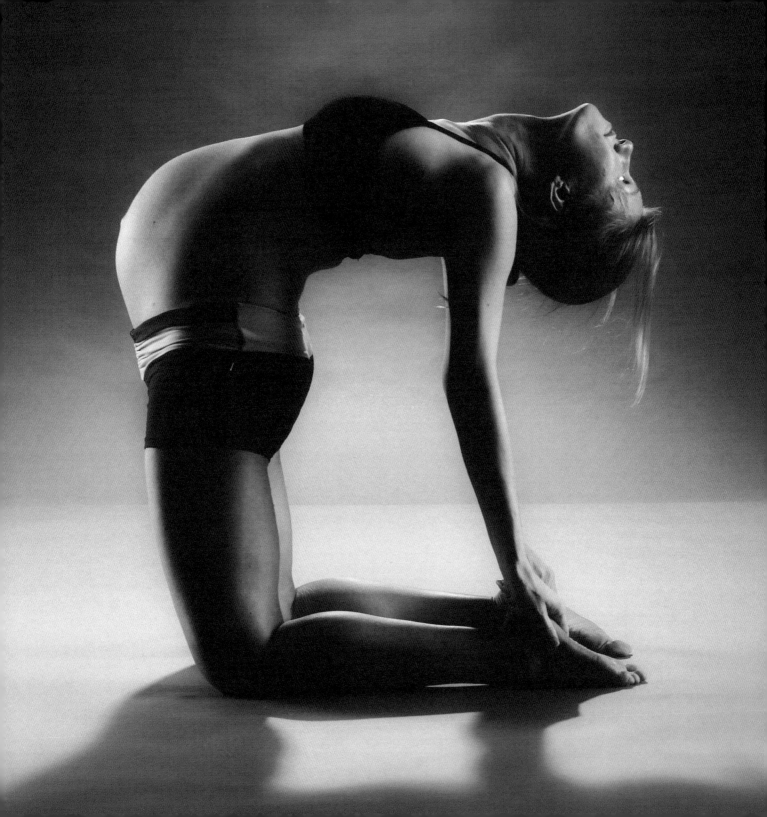

> It was five weeks after birth when I returned to yoga class. By ten weeks post-birth, I was only five pounds more than my pre-pregnancy weight.

I had never truly given myself that permission before. I have since incorporated this into my practice, and I realize that this is just the beginning of a path of absorbing more and more benefits available to me through yoga. I am learning to let go of what I should be able to do in a posture and accept where I am. In being present, I usually find that I can go deeper into a pose.

Another benefit I learned during my pregnancy was to conserve energy. I became conscious of all the extra movements in my practice and eliminated many of them. Carrying around that extra weight was enough extra work. Did I really need to bring a washcloth to wipe off my perspiration? No. Did I need to fix my hair after half moon? No. Did I need to drink water every time after eagle pose? No. Conserving energy allowed me to participate in all the postures (with some modifications, obviously), even when I was two days away from giving birth. I did not have to sit out many postures in my second and third trimesters.

Another non-physical aspect to my practice was the sense of community at my studio. As my body changed, people noticed, and everyone was enthusiastic and excited for me. And they were encouraging, too. It made me happy to be there. I loved being in front of the mirror, watching my body as it changed, and I think others did, too. It was fun how others noticed that how my baby was growing. It did not make me self-conscious; it made me feel proud and grateful that my body was growing a baby. I appreciated all the kind words.

Going through this life-changing experience and having a sense of community is important. I am lucky to have a wonderful husband, a terrific family, and a good circle of friends, but the sense of community I found at my studio added a another dimension. It was a place to get away from my daily life. I practiced alongside mothers, fathers, sisters, brothers, aunts, and uncles. Their support and different perspectives made me appreciate the excitement of being pregnant.

When I started the modifications, I was lucky to have other pregnant teachers around to guide me. Each pregnant woman had her own way of modifying the practice, but the goal was always to make room for the baby in the poses: Don't compress the belly. Jordin Murphree spent the most time with me and was always eager to answer any of my questions. I developed my own set of modifications that felt right for me and for my body. And those modifications evolved as my belly grew.

One of the best benefits to doing yoga when I was pregnant was the connection I developed to Ethan. There were several times that I could actually see him move when I was looking in the mirror! It was such an amazing feeling. And I always had a little internal conversation with him during the moments on the floor at the end of the class. On the days I didn't do yoga, the only quiet times I truly had to do this was right before I fell asleep. And that was always at the end of an exhausting day. In yoga, it may have been at the end of an exhausting class, but I always feel so alive at the end of class with all that blood and oxygen pulsing through my body. It was a great time to "talk" to my son.

Birth felt like something I went through with Ethan. I felt like we were a team (along with my husband, who was nothing short of amazing). Feeling that connection to Ethan helped me during labor. Yoga isn't the only way to feel a connection with your baby, but it is a great way.

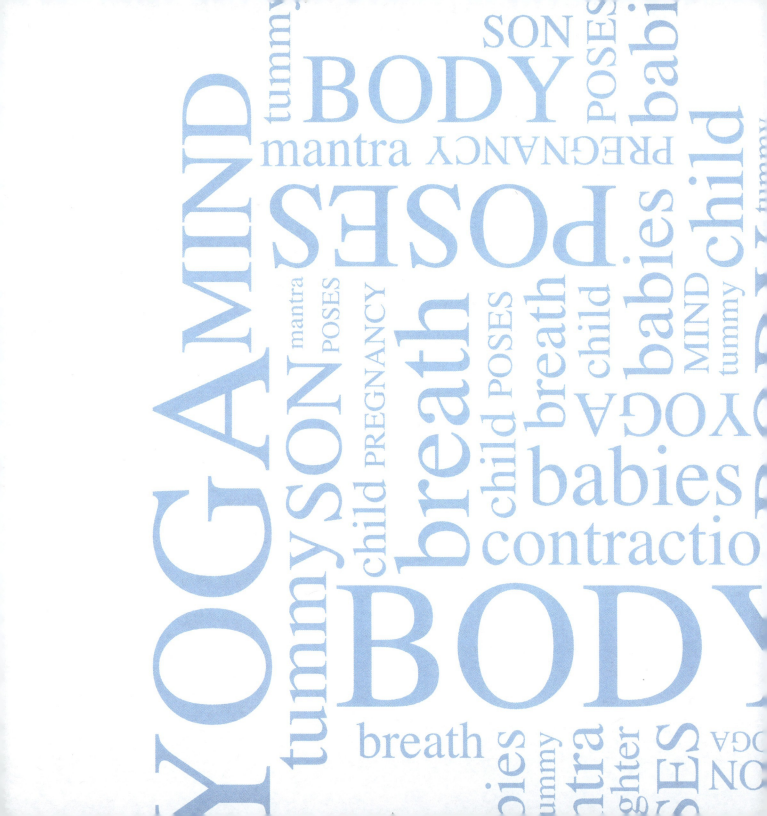

YOGA PREGNANCY babies breath breath breath mantra babies contractions MIND child SON MIND POSES mantra contractions SON contractions babies daughter MIND

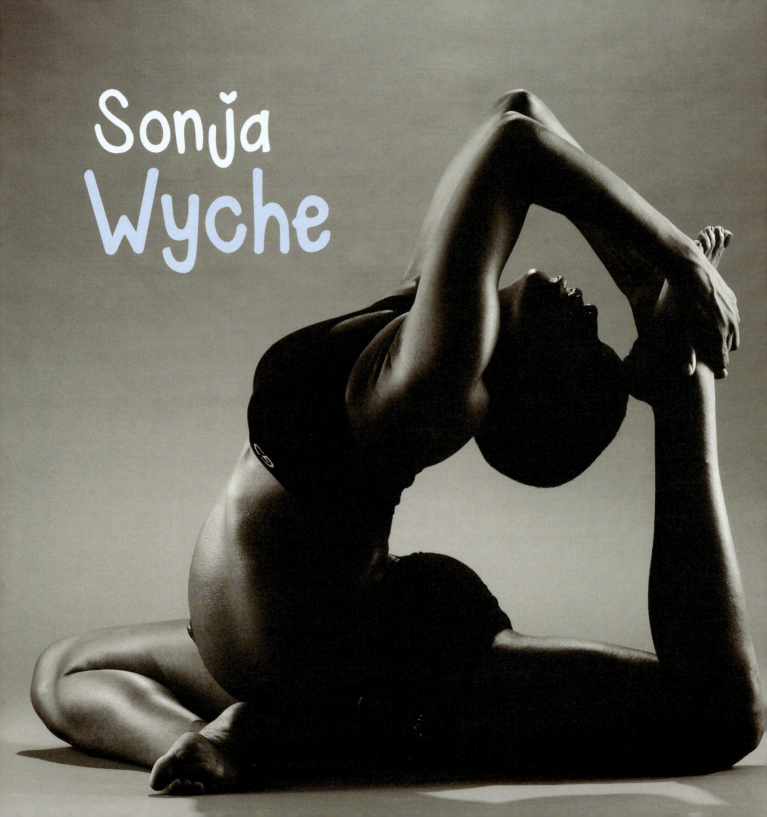
Sonja Wyche

I never had a hard time getting pregnant, and I guess that is why I just assumed that my transition from a yogi to a pregnant yogi would be easy. I found out I was pregnant with Monroe on December 17, 2008, one day after taking a yoga posture clinic. I remember it all so vividly. I had just participated in a yoga demonstration. It was a joyous moment to be able to express the asanas with my fellow yogis.

As I told more and more people about my wonderful pregnancy, congratulations always accompanied warnings of, "I hope you aren't going to still do that yoga. You know you have to be careful and take it easy—you are pregnant now." I could understand caution but this was evoking fear. I would say to myself, "I know that I am pregnant, but I feel fine."

I went on living the way I always had, trusting that my body would naturally prepare me for the life growing inside of me. With a smooth transition, my body changed: My muscles softened, and my once flat-as-a-board stomach slowly poked out and rounded ever so softly. I would find myself resting my hands on my belly. And, yes, I was still practicing yoga. Or, better yet, the yoga was practicing me. I soon found myself benefiting from yoga more than I ever had before.

When I awoke and felt like crying, when my clothes didn't fit, when my back hurt because I slept wrong, I practiced yoga. It forced me to stop running and look at myself, and I loved me as a result. I would breathe deeply and let it all out, and soon I'd be relaxed. With each inhale and exhale, I'd hear the instructor slowly counting to six; my shoulders would let go, my neck was no longer stiff, the aches in my back would go away, and the tingling sensation in my toes and feet would disappear. Sometimes I wondered if my fellow yogis looked at me and questioned it. "Why is she in class? She could be hurting the child growing inside her." Or, "Why is she doing the postures differently?" The modified postures are important while pregnant because your center of gravity changes. Doing the modifications allowed me to stay in balance while practicing during my pregnancy.

I had been practicing, and things were smooth. I was a pregnant yogi, and I accepted it. Then I went to my first OB appointment. Needless to say, fear was at the top of my list. I stood on the scale, my blood pressure was checked, and everything was positive. The doctor came in, we shared pleasantries and I had my first sonogram. My OB encouraged me to exercise regularly, but not excessively and to keep it to about 30 minutes daily. I replied, "Are you serious?!"

I told her about my yoga practice, and she was silent. She gave me the stare-down and warned me that I could potentially harm my baby and that I shouldn't do it. "What is so bad about the practice and pregnancy?" I asked. I was on the verge of tears because yoga was keeping me in balance, and I didn't want her to take my practice away. I knew what I felt in my heart and body. I could feel the response I got from my growing child when I practiced. When I'd go through the half moon series, I'd giggle as my baby bulge shifted from side to side, and little parts started poking out and moving all around. These moments reminded me how right all this was for me.

I was really into my practice throughout my pregnancy. I could see my body changing and was getting comfortable with the fact that I had to put the skinny jeans in the back of my closet. I felt great when I'd go to my regular OB visits and hear that my blood pressure was great, there was no swelling in my legs, and my weight gain was appropriate and on schedule. Maybe some mothers take these things for granted, but keep in my mind that when pregnant, not only are you changing on the outside, but the physiologic changes going on inside your body are overwhelming as well. Every organ, blood vessel, and cell in a mother's body must work together to carry the growing child.

With exercise, most especially yoga, the body is in constant motion and releases endorphins, allowing blood vessels to relax and increase blood flow not just through mommy's body, but also in the baby's, delivering important nutrients and oxygen. Yoga practice also regulates weight gain, decreasing the risk of macrosomia (a large gestational baby). This condition can bring complications such as gestational diabetes. Also with a large baby, you also challenges during delivery. Large babies sometimes require scheduled C-sections instead of normal deliveries.

I was so pleased to be on the "right track." With pregnancy, my center of gravity changed constantly, but yoga kept me well-balanced, especially with the half moon series. One of my favorites was balancing stick posture, where I just let my belly hang and extended my arms and legs in opposite directions. Many friends complained of back pain throughout their pregnancies and of sciatica, which is when the sciatic nerve becomes impinged in the vertebral column, causing severe pain down the back of the leg. This condition is often really debilitating. I needed the movement, the daily flow. It kept my joints flushed, my body open and my mind free. I had no back pain whatsoever.

So then came the bombshell: I went for my five-month sonogram and was told by the radiologist that there is an abnormality in my baby's brain. I didn't even listen to the explanations. All I heard was that something was not right, not normal. I immediately started to wonder if it was due to the yoga. Did I bend incorrectly, or was it the heat in the yoga room? I was taking my temperature at every class and never went above 99°F. What was it? Why wasn't everything right and normal? I went home and just cried—cried for everything. I remembered feeling my belly and just knowing that it would all be OK, no matter the outcome, and I also reassured myself that I was doing the best that I could do.

I needed the yoga now more than ever. Pranayama breathing became deeper, longer, and refreshing, cleansing my mind of negative thoughts. Savasana was my alone time with my baby when I would feel a lot of movement and was reminded of my miracle. My practice got me through the uncertainty and made me feel strong.

I practiced almost daily throughout pregnancy and felt blessed every day to be able to do so. When I knew my delivery day was rapidly approaching I was nervous and excited at the same time. On August 15, 2009, when I was 39 weeks pregnant, I practiced at the 4 p.m. class. It was a good class, and I jokingly said I wished this class would put me in labor (the power of thought).

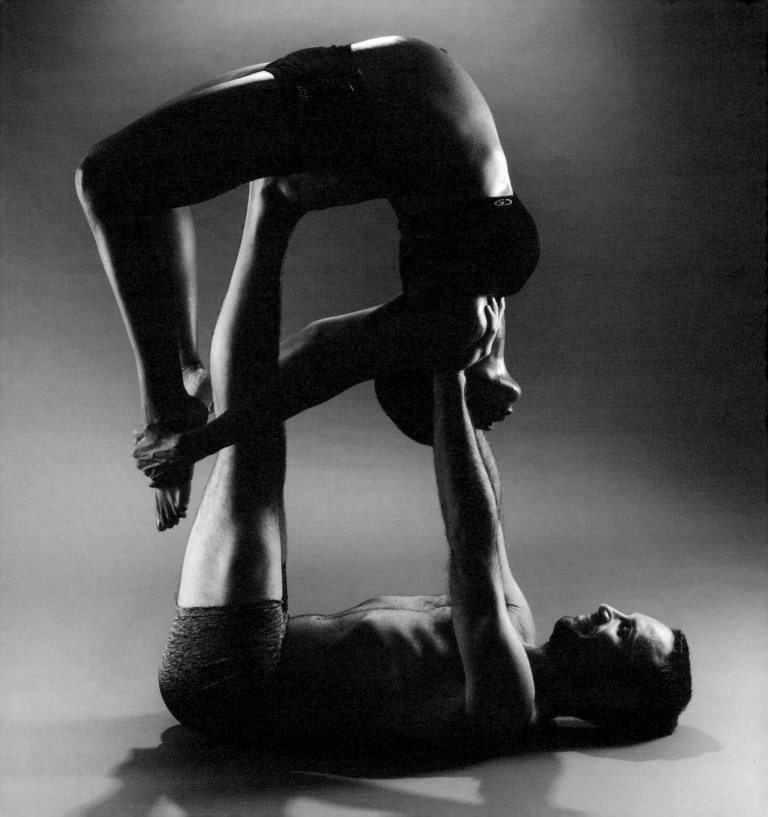

Lo and behold, my water broke, and the contractions started later on that evening. in the early morning hours of August 16, 2009, my husband and I welcomed our perfectly healthy little princess, Monroe Evan. Everything was smooth and safe, and there were no abnormalities in her brain. I also have to let you know that I was up and about one day later.

What will I take with me from this experience? I love myself. Yoga has taught me to accept the transitions that life brings. Yoga brought me closer to my growing baby. It felt so good to exercise, to give my baby a wonderful gift of peace. The exercise did not put stress or strain on my body—no high impact—but it definitely got my heart pumping and blood flowing. The sweating released toxins while cooling my body simultaneously. Yoga will always be a part of my life and my family's life. It helped me to be in balance throughout my pregnancy.

Pregnancy is a time of transformation and many transitions. It is so important to keep a constant yoga practice in this time of change. Just breathe. Remember when all the challenges surround you, when people stare and question your intentions, just tell them, "I'm pregnant, people, not dead!" Movement is not just important—it is essential.

As I am bending backwards, stretching, or even taking deep breaths, I have asked myself, why yoga? Why when I am pregnant? Shouldn't I be worried? Is it safe? What about the baby? Is it fair to the baby? Shouldn't I be taking it easy? Should I fold my legs? And when my doctor tells me to get 30 minutes of exercise a day, does it include yoga? Have you ever thought about why it is important to exercise at all? And why it's so important to exercise when pregnant?

Do you understand what pregnancy does to the body? You gain at least 20 pounds, so your bones are carrying around extra weight, and your back has to hold that weight up. Your heart goes into workout mode and pumps more blood throughout your body. You deal with swelling, or pooling of blood, around your ankles and feet. Hormones are bouncing around your body, and your mood fluctuates constantly. Your ligaments and joints have increased laxity. Oh, and even digestion changes: more indigestion, constipation, and nausea from hormones and prenatal vitamins.

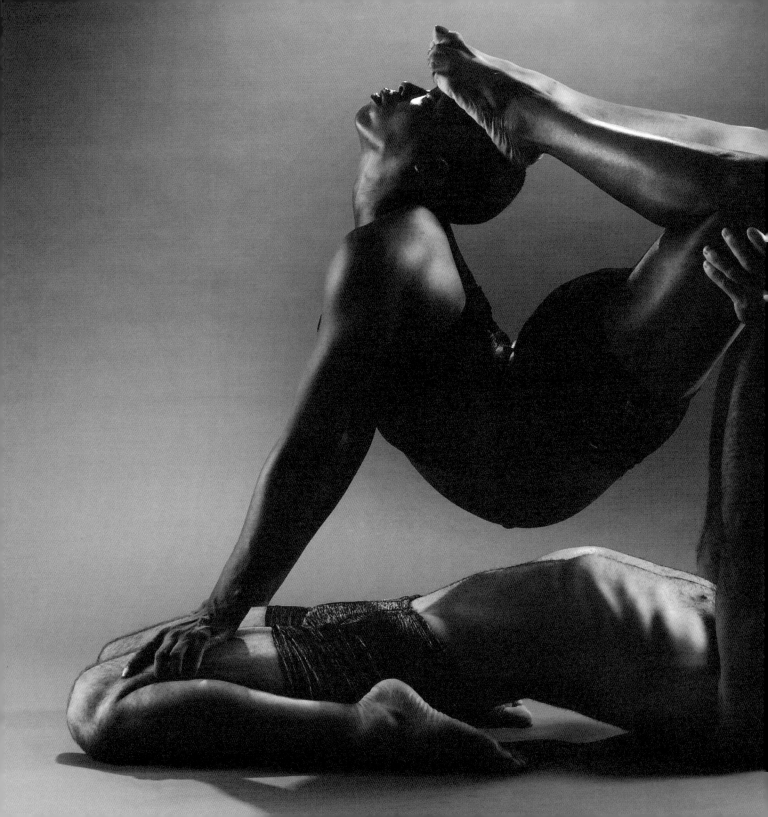

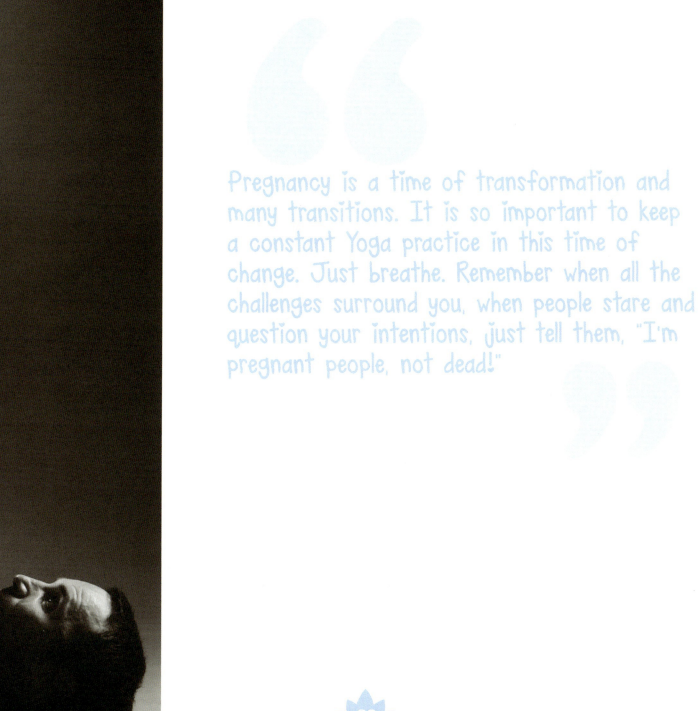

"Pregnancy is a time of transformation and many transitions. It is so important to keep a constant Yoga practice in this time of change. Just breathe. Remember when all the challenges surround you, when people stare and question your intentions, just tell them, "I'm pregnant people, not dead!"

Despite the pensive stares, or the repetitive question, "Are you sure it's OK for you to stretch like that during pregnancy?" I always responded with, "This is the best time to stretch. There's no other time that it's more important than when you are pregnant." I can't think of any other exercise that gives back what you put into it; yoga has been around for thousands of years. It's so consistent. The yoga community is so supportive and allows you to just be and receive love and support from others all in the same room doing the same thing. There is no banging music, no jarring movements—just flowing, just being, and just feeling. Feeling each and every movement in my body gives me energy, allows me to release all of my frustrations, fears and challenges and at the same time fueling my body and being with truth and love.

My favorite posture has always been standing bow. I raise one arm way up into the air and toward the sky. I kick my other leg up and away, and I look at myself in the mirror, and I see a beautiful person. My swollen belly pokes out and drops with me as I open up.

I didn't find yoga. This practice found me, and it corrects me daily. So when a pregnant woman approaches me and asks if it is OK to practice yoga, I ask her if she wants to give her growing child the best gift ever: nourishment, strength, and health. Practicing yoga while pregnant strengthens your back (remember, we only have one), opens pores, helps flush the body and sends blood everywhere, balances metabolism, and keeps hormones in check. As women, we are blessed with the ability to bring life into this world. Why not try to be the best vessel possible for that growing child?

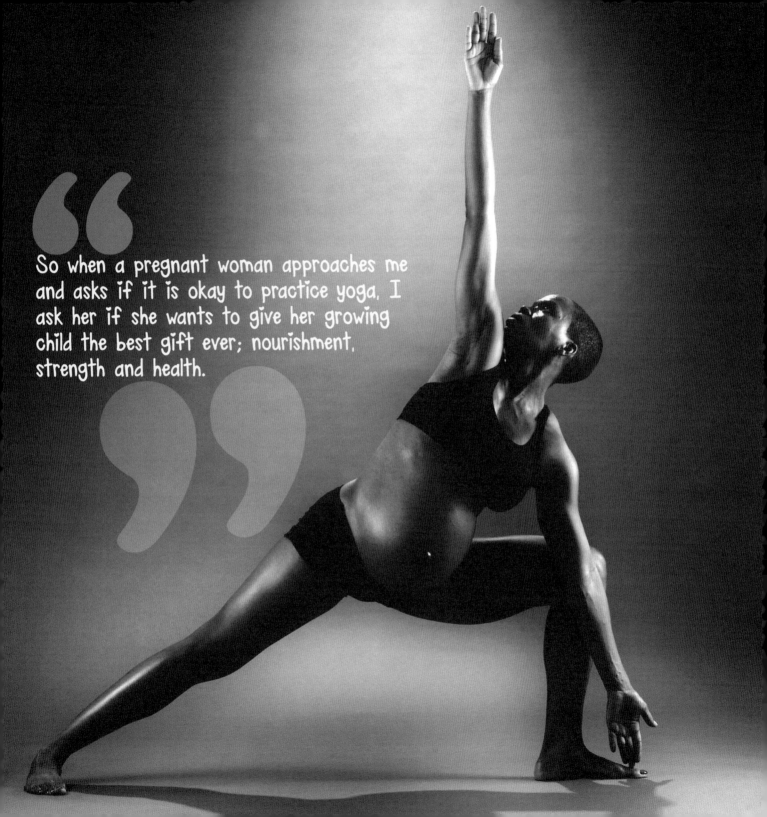

> So when a pregnant woman approaches me and asks if it is okay to practice yoga, I ask her if she wants to give her growing child the best gift ever; nourishment, strength and health.

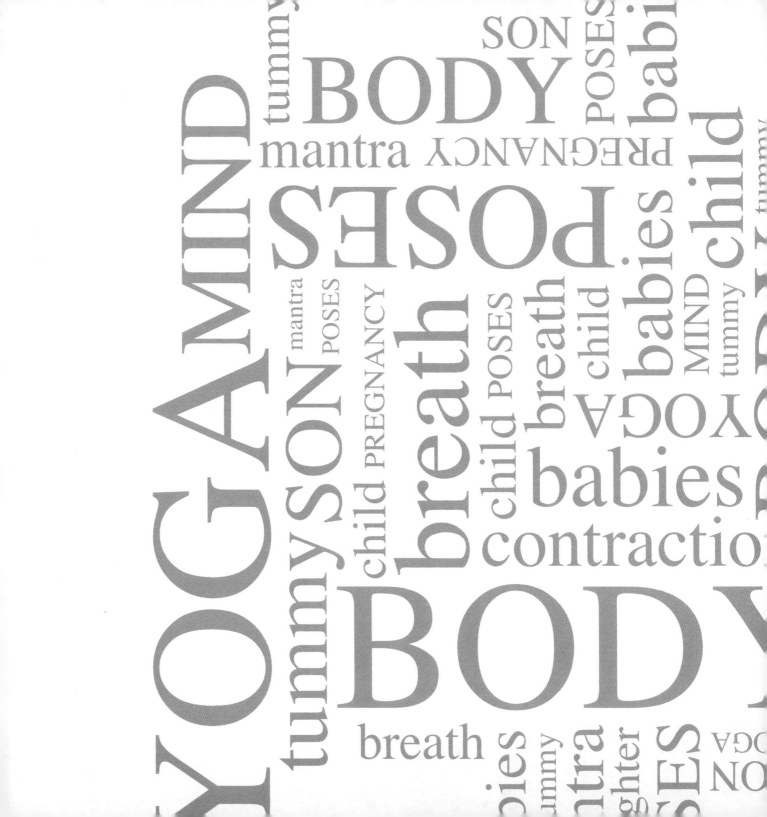

mantra breath babies contractions breath YOGA breath PREGNANCY SON babies child MIND contractions daughter MIND mmy SON MIND POSES mantra contractions

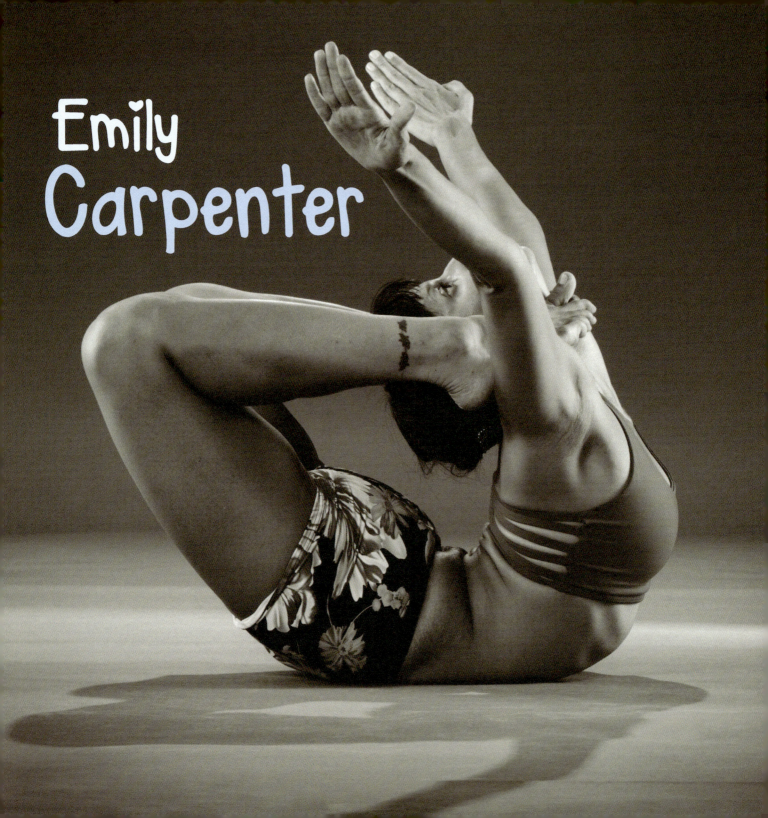

Everyone's birth experience is different. I've heard and read a lot of different stories and none have ever been quite the same. Having said that, I think that knowing about different women and their experiences with pregnancy and labor can really help in those moments when you just want to give up. When I became pregnant with my daughter Juliana, I had been practicing yoga for eight years. Yoga had led me to become the most active I had ever been. I was facing my fear of heights and rock climbing and skiing better than ever! When I became pregnant and had to modify a lot of my activities, having my practice stay consistent was very helpful.

When I became pregnant, my husband and I were doing some home remodeling. I noticed my tastes changing and my boobs getting bigger and more tender, but I did not realize that pregnancy was the reason. I became very sensitive to the smell of chemicals and could not bring myself to do the painting that I had committed to. After a very emotional fight over why my end of the project wasn't done, I decided that I needed to go get a pregnancy test. I guess I don't need to state the obvious, but I got the plus sign.

I am a hot yoga teacher, and I was scheduled to teach at one of the studios my husband and I own. My husband was a champion, and he covered my classes for the next couple of days while I found a doctor and adjusted to the idea that I had a baby inside of me. Hot yoga really speaks to my heart, and a regular practice keeps me balanced both physically and emotionally. With my first baby, I was told not to practice while pregnant because the heat of the room would raise my body temperature. I decided to test this theory, and I took my temperature after a few classes. To my surprise, it didn't change at all, so I kept practicing about three times a week. My husband's mom, who is a doctor, gave me some great ideas about how to modify my practice. Pregnancy made me feel ill for most of my first trimester, so I took it easy, and what little I was able to do felt like a big accomplishment.

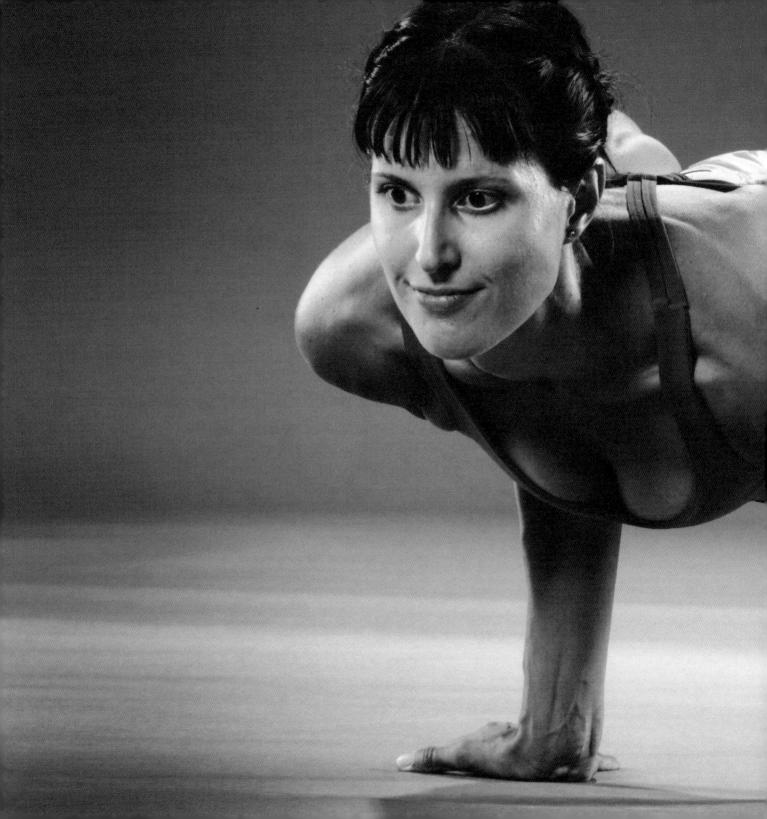

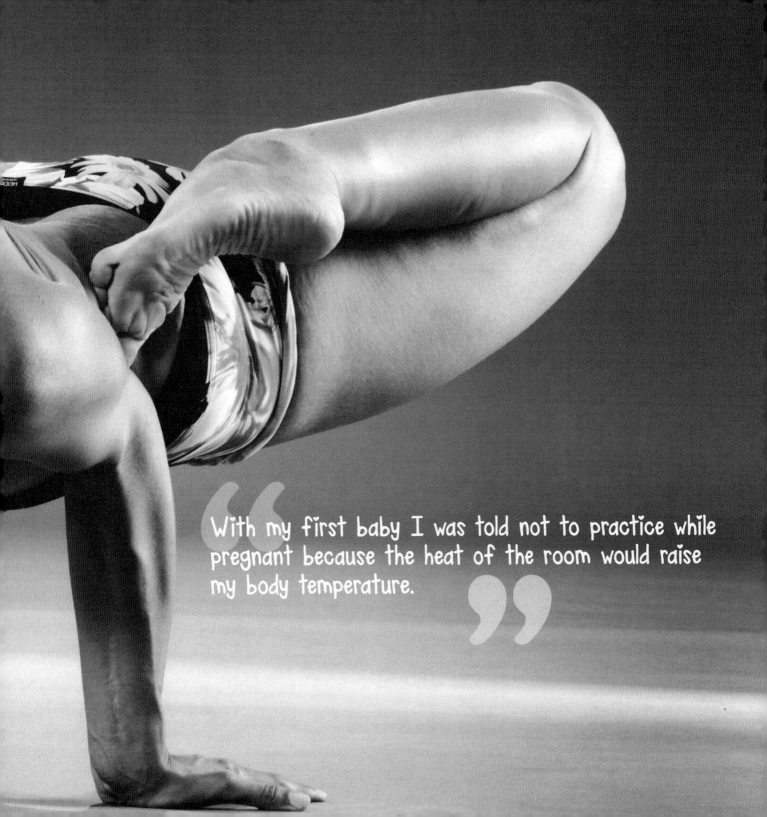

" With my first baby I was told not to practice while pregnant because the heat of the room would raise my body temperature. "

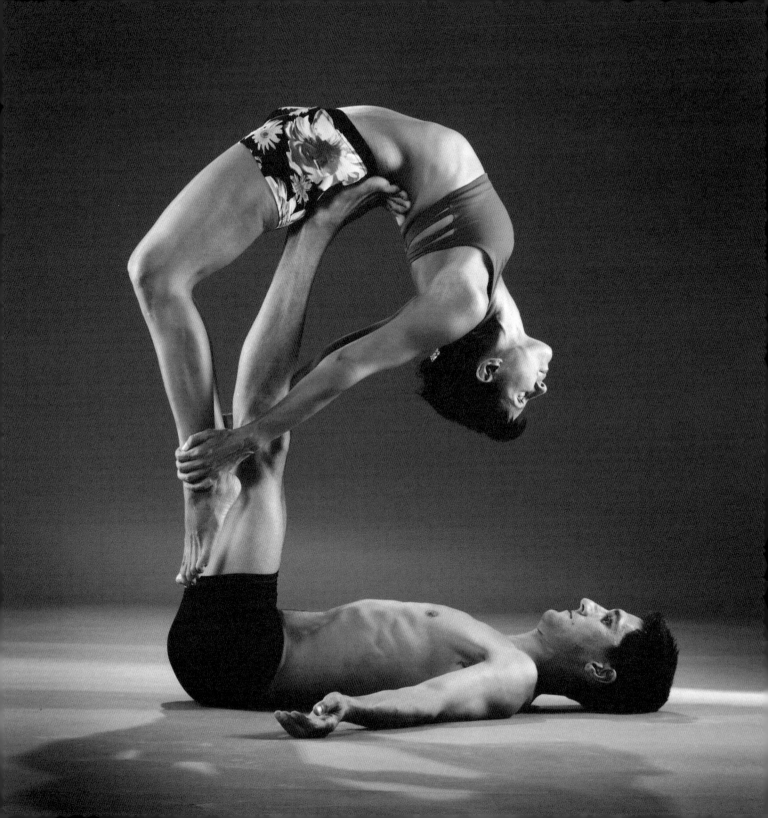

After the first three months there was a switch, and all of a sudden I had more energy. I wasn't so sensitive to smells, and I was finally able get a good sweat going. It felt like my body had adjusted to being pregnant. I found a wonderful doctor who understood that yoga was my lifestyle and that not practicing would be more dangerous to my health than simply keeping it up. I kept practicing three to four times a week until a few months later when I saw Bikram and Rajashree. They both gave me so much encouragement and support that I started practicing every day until the day before Juliana was born.

Rajashree's pregnancy series, a modified version of the regular practice, kept me feeling strong and so healthy. I loved going to the studio and watching my baby get bigger in the mirror. The students loved seeing my belly in the postures, and I would have students come up and tell me that they could see the baby moving when we were in savasana. We all became closer, and I felt a lot of love and support.

Juliana was a week late; I felt like she was never going to come. I tried to induce labor by being more active than usual, even turning over the garden, but nothing would break my water, so I decided to let my doctor do it. I wanted to have natural birth, but that sack was not going to open on its own.

Your birth plan is special; it's your vision, but it is also important to be flexible because anything can happen, and the more relaxed you stay, the better it is for you and your baby. My practice taught me to be in control of my mind and body. I think it is amazing that in the practice, you can be balancing on one leg with the muscles on one side of your body contracted, and the muscles on the opposite side of your body completely relaxed. Through yoga I learned how to know my body and how to trust it. I labored with Juliana for a little over 10 hours, which isn't very long in the scheme of things, but it felt like a long time while it was happening. I had a lot of back labor (pain in my lower back) so I stayed on my feet and knees when things got really intense. I had done some hypnosis that helped to keep my subconscious clean and calm, even when the person in the room next to me was screaming her head off.

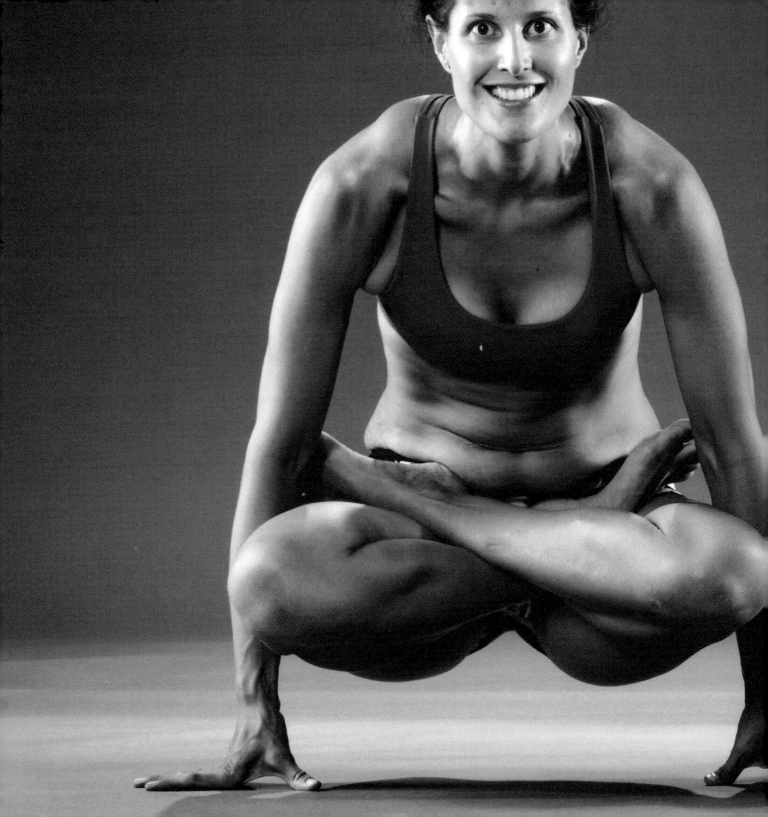

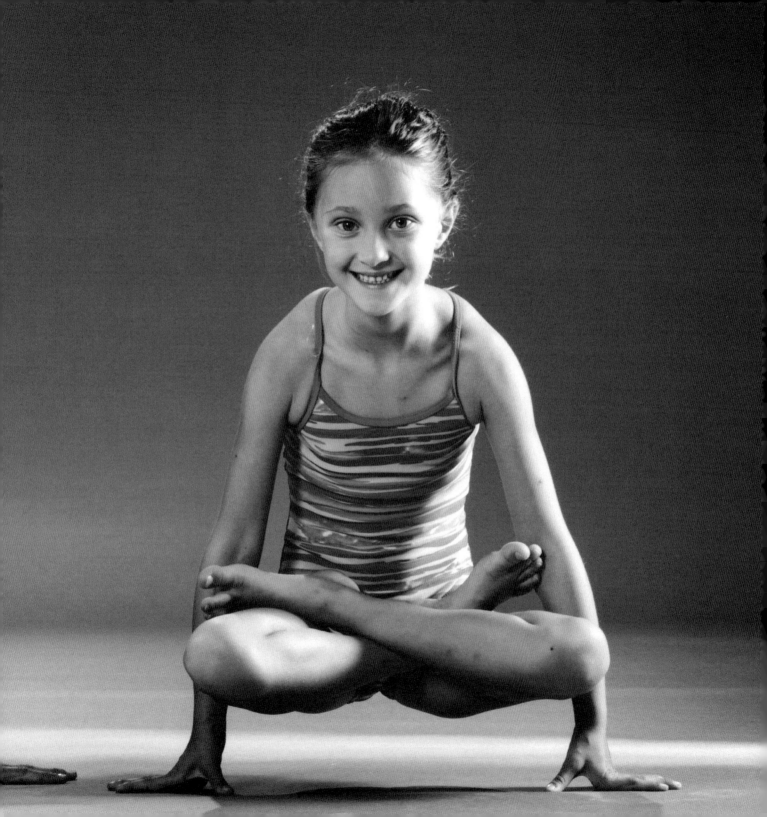

I think women all have a vision of how we want our labor to go. When you visualize yours, it really helps to see that end moment when you're holding your baby in your arms. When I reached nine centimeters, my mom and my mother-in-law came in and assisted in the delivery. I felt like the team I needed was there, and now we were ready to go. My mom was on my left, my husband was on my right, and my mother-in-law supported the rhythm of my contractions and guided me through the pushes and pauses of labor. Towards the end, I rounded forward like in rabbit pose, and as I pushed my daughter out, I was actually able to watch everything happen. I think because of all the sweating and stretching I did in yoga, I didn't tear and was able to bounce back quickly. I went back to yoga 10 days after having my daughter, who was 7 lbs., 4 oz., and I went skiing the day after that. Going back to yoga really helped me when I was starting to feel some irrational emotions like in post-postpartum depression. In the yoga practice, you observe your thoughts, feelings, and physical sensations. Eventually, you get used to doing this in your everyday life as well, and it helps you stay rational and keep emotions in check.

Having my daughter has taught me so much about myself and my own unresolved issues. It reminded me that I need to take care of myself, because if I don't, then who's going to take care of my kids?! My second pregnancy didn't go quite as smoothly as my first. I think that I got a bit of a big head about having babies after having a relatively easy time with Juliana. When my husband and I decided to go for number two, he wanted to start right away, but I wasn't feeling it yet, and that created some friction. Once I was ready, we conceived almost immediately.

This time, I kept practicing hot yoga regularly, and a yoga day felt so much better than a non-yoga day. I maintained a lot of my deeper postures and gained only 25 pounds instead of the 50 lbs I gained my first time around. I also kept on teaching, and, of course, took care of my daughter.

It was a challenging time because my husband became very passionate about opening another studio, and I wanted to focus on our family. We struggled with finding a balance between our family and work responsibilities, and my life was feeling a little bumpy when I went in for my five-month check up. We went to the doctor to find out the sex of the baby and learned that not only were we having a boy, but also that the baby was breech and I had placenta previa (when the placenta grows over the cervical opening).

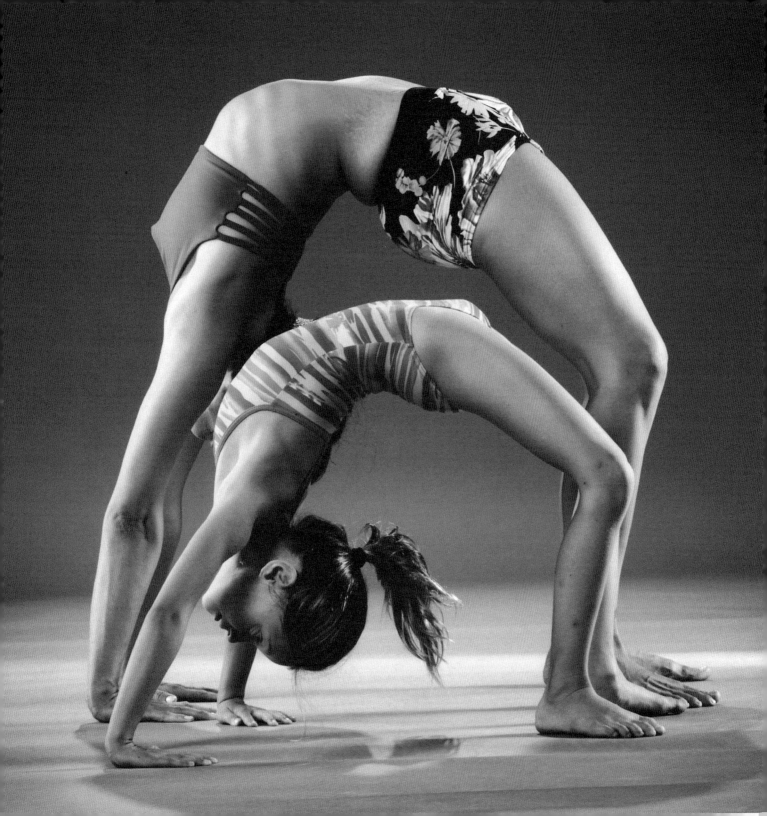

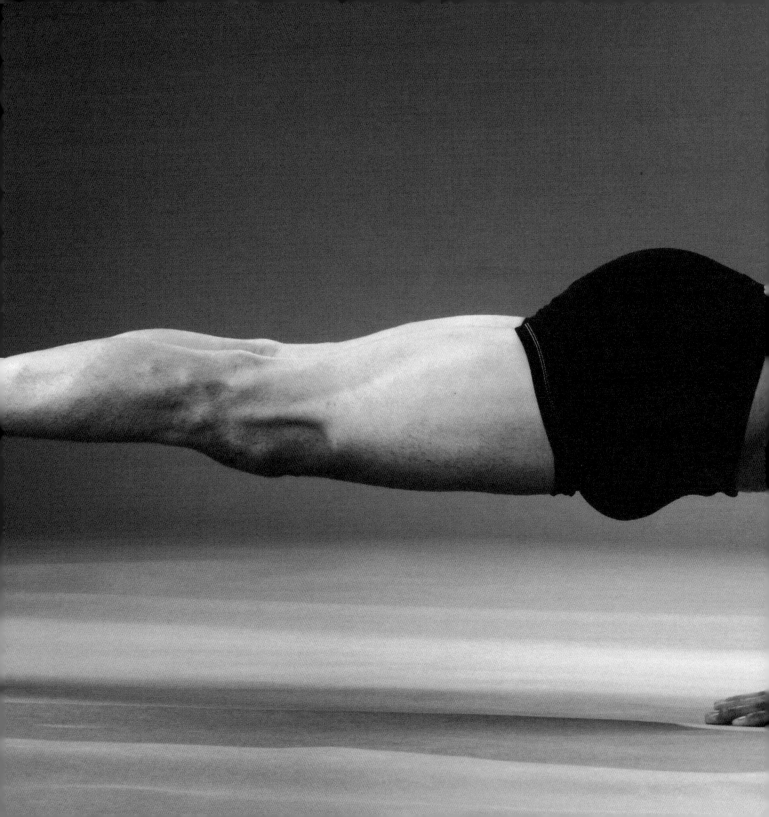

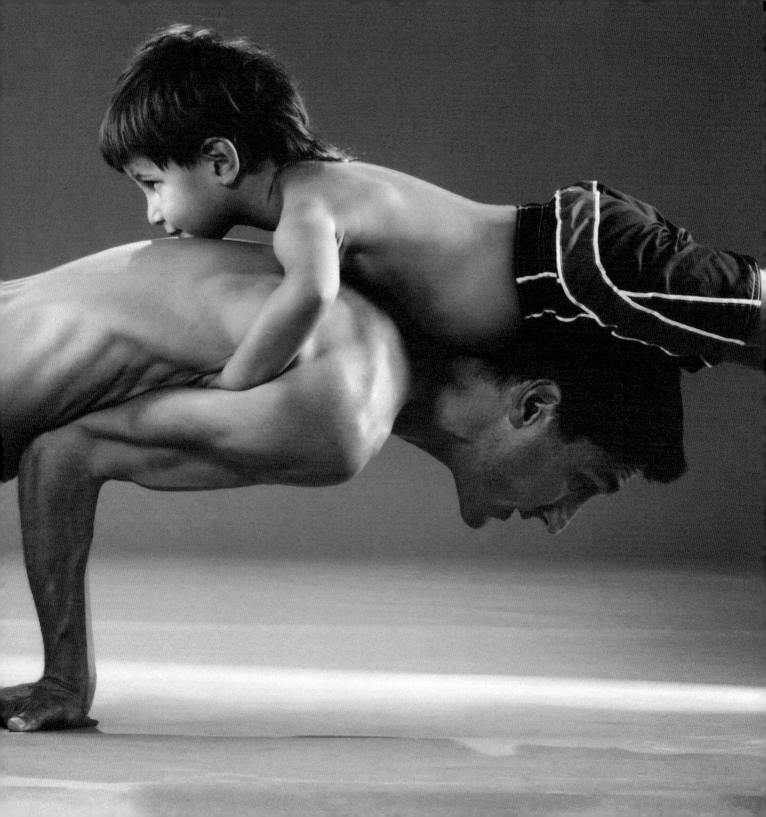

The doctor informed me that if the baby didn't turn, and if my placenta didn't move away from my cervix, then I would have to get a C-section. I felt like I was in a bad dream. Thank God Juliana came to the appointment, or I may have totally lost it on the spot. How was I going to take care of a three-year-old and newborn after stomach surgery? I did not want any needles near my back! I wanted a home birth, and with a C-section that was not a possibility. I kept telling myself that this wasn't my karma or baby Soren's. I remembered that in my birthing class they had shown me postures just like the floor modifications in Rajashree's pregnancy class, so I started to focus on those moves and looked to other alternatives to remedy my situation. I did acupuncture, cranial sacral hypnosis, and my daily yoga practice. When I went in for my next checkup and found that nothing had changed, I was devastated and felt like giving up. Doing yoga felt hard; why was I working so much when they were just going to cut me open? Why hadn't anything worked yet?

Slowly, I began to realize that we can't control our births. I had been lucky to have had such an easy time with my first child, but in the end, having a healthy baby was more important than how the baby came out. I realized that I was worried that not going through with natural childbirth would reflect poorly on me and my philosophy on health and living. Wow. I was doing some heavy-duty growing so I decided to start talking about my situation and my fears instead of denying them.

The yoga community was very supportive, and there was no judgment. Friends were concerned and offered assistance if I needed it. They didn't think that I was any less of a person, and they didn't think that my yoga practice had caused this situation. I was suddenly filled with admiration for all of the women that needed assistance with their deliveries and so grateful for modern technology. With a more open mind, I went back to work doing what I could but with less attachment. When Juliana and I went in for my seven-month check up on Halloween, I made sure not to get my hopes up. The visit started as usual. Juliana was in her Wonder Woman costume which was very comforting to me because that was always my favorite superhero.

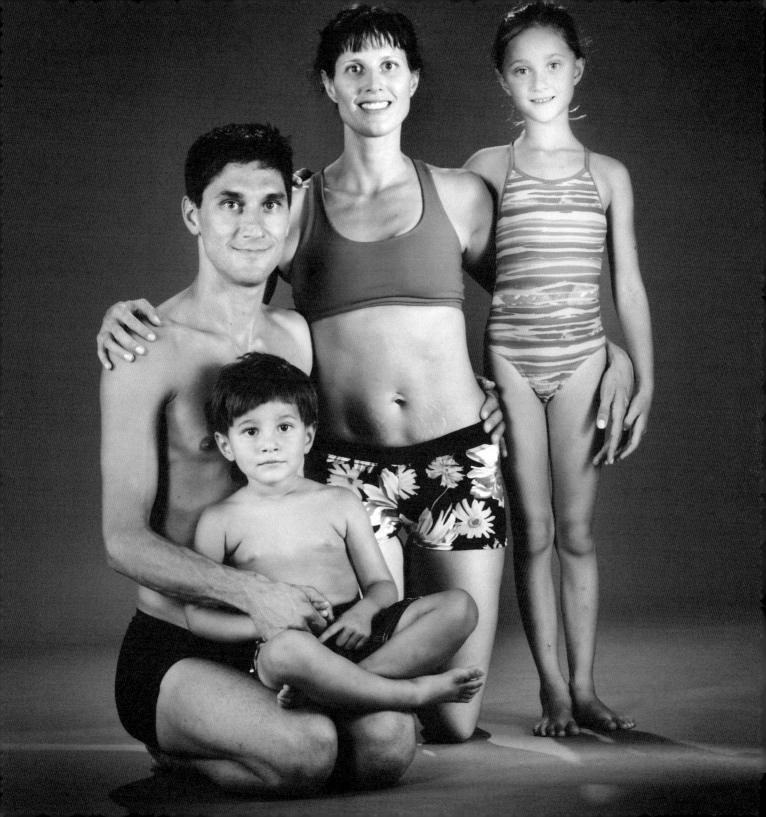

As my doctor was probing around with the ultrasound, she suddenly got excited, and when she was sure of what she saw, she told me the good news. The baby had not only turned into a normal position, but he had also moved the placenta off my cervix. I couldn't believe that we were in the clear! Before all these complications, I had been contemplating having a home birth, and now that everything was back to normal, I had to re-evaluate my ideal birthing plan. Every time I thought of home, it just didn't feel right. I loved the relationship I had with my doctor, and I knew she respected my wishes. I respected her knowledge and skill and trusted if my body wasn't up to it or if the baby was in distress, she would step in and help get me through. She also respected my wish to have my husband deliver the baby and to have my mom and mother-in-law be involved.

About a month before my due date, I started to dilate so I took it easy for a week but quickly realized that, like Juliana, this baby wanted to take his time. Once again, my due date passed with no baby appearing. The waiting was the worst. I would go to yoga, and everyone would tell me that they would give me their towels if I went into labor. The good thing about the second time around is you know it doesn't happen that fast, and that you will probably have time to get to your desired birth place.

A week after my due date, my doctor and I talked about breaking my water. I was hoping we wouldn't have to do it, but the longer we waited, the more dangerous it would be for the baby. I had a feeling that it was time, and we decided to meet on a Saturday. This gave me enough time to get my mother-in-law, my mom, and my husband all together. My dad took care of Juliana and our animals so I could finally relax and have this baby.

During both labors, I was so blessed to have great nurses who gave me tips which helped to keep things moving. My first nurse told me to pant like a dog whenever I had back labor! I'm sure this sounds crazy, but it keeps you from pushing until you're 10 centimeters dilated. It also prevents your cervix from getting as swollen, so you can push and relax your baby out with less pain and less tearing. My second nurse noticed that when my daughter was around my contractions would stop, so she helped me delegate and had my dad take Juliana out. I really wanted Juliana there, but in retrospect, I think it would have been too much for her.

Once she was gone, my body got with the program, and contractions came regularly. Most of my water was in the upper part of the amniotic sac, and my baby's head was blocking it from coming out. This is why his pressure wasn't breaking the sac. In order to get all the water out, my second nurse made me do figure eights with my hips while leaning on the bed. This also positioned the baby so when I reached 10 centimeters, we would be ready.

I found that during both labors, about every hour or so, I would glance at the clock and something about this kept me on track and helped me manage my pain. It felt like yoga class, when the intense moments of an asana are followed by the calm of savasana.

When they told me to push, I was timid at first and nothing happened. At that moment, I realized that I was the director this time, and instead of just trying to manage pain and let the birth happen, I was going to have to take charge and really push this baby out. I needed to stay active, and I ended up standing, squatting, and doing figure eights with my hips for more than three hours. I was glad for the stamina I had developed in the standing series of hot yoga and felt that without that training, I would have given up. I ended up laboring for about six hours. My mom and nurse took my legs this time, and my mother-in-law held down my perineum, which helps to prevent tearing. As I pushed my baby out, my husband held and guided him. He was the first one to touch Soren, and it was both a magical and strenuous time. It is a moment I can still go back to and see clearly, like a picture.

I loved bringing the family together for the births of both my children. It made us all closer, and I feel like each person helped me make it through those challenging moments. Without my yoga practice, I wouldn't have known and trusted my body enough to go through two deliveries with minimal medical intervention. After having my son, I started practicing five days after getting my doctor's approval. Boy, did I ever feel ready to have my own practice again. I had to leave early when my milk let down to feed the baby, but I instantly started feeling more like myself, and it helped me to manage my emotions, my recovery, and my bigger family.

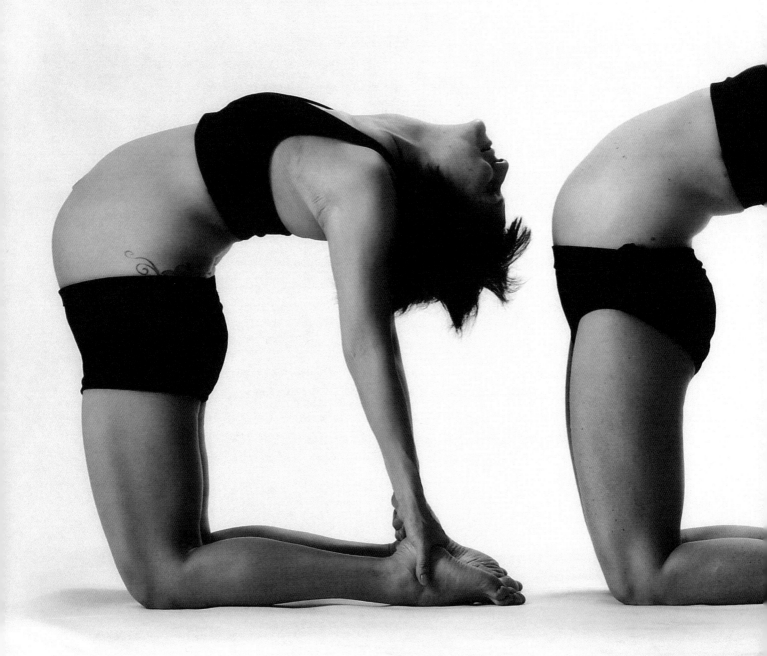

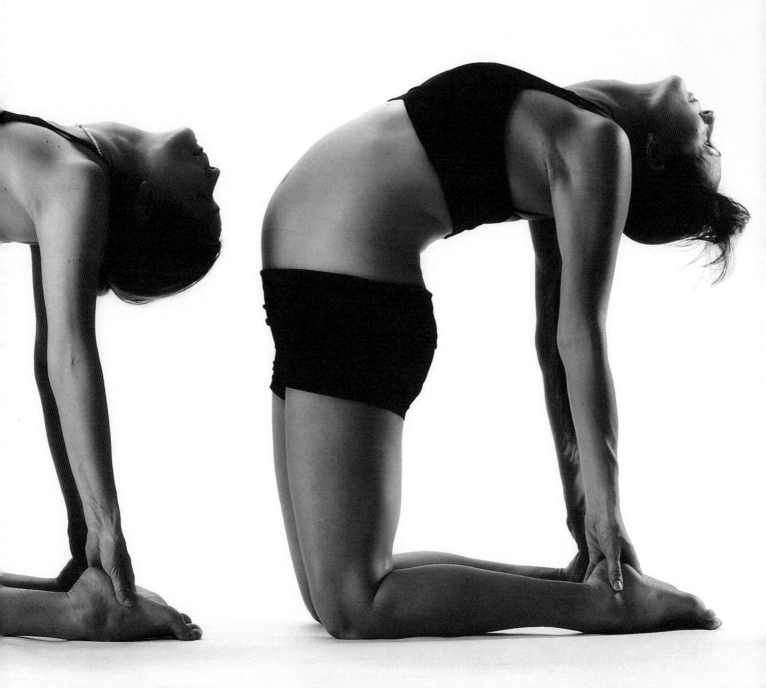

Thank You

Thank you to the mamas in this book who have inspired so many in their respective studios. With love for the beings they carried in their wombs, they have continued their practices in a compassionate way.

I had a wonderful crew of friends assist me in this book. I'd like to thank Dan Knudson for donating these wonderful pictures and helping the women in the book feel very comfortable during every shoot. When I met Dan, I told him about the book and mentioned that I did not have much money in my budget for travel, so I hoped that many yoginis became pregnant in Boulder, Colorado, (where Dan resides). Months later, five of the yoginis in this book became pregnant!

Especially thank you to Mary Jarvis. Observing Mary guide mothers to be in the "little orange room" at Global Yoga in San Francisco was a big inspiration for this book. Thank you Mary! Thank you to my Capoeira Angola Mestre Cobra Mansa for keeping sharing capoeira and giving me a place that is home.

Also I wish to thank Brian Keith of KarmaSavvy.com for reformatting the book and putting it online for people to access. To Yassi Maige, Insel Metin, Kelly Schrader, Alex & Jackie Wheeler, Bronek Gacki, Jonny & Amber Mauk, Esak Garcia, Liz & Anthony Cotter, Lizzie Clark, Lisa Ingle, Maryam Ovissi, Meghan Huehn, Alexandra Evans, Andrew Byey, Rusty Wells, The Urban Flow Tribe and many other friends for giving me a home during my travels and a space to share the Synergy Partner Yoga practice.

Thank you to the yoga studio owners Radha Garcia and Rima "Nation" Hinnawi for sharing their studios for the photo shoots. To Rosario de Lavalle, Little Aspen Ali, Ipek Davaz, and chunks for editing the text from a jumble of words into something easy to read.

Thank you to the teachers who continue to share the wonderment of yoga with many. To my mother Marita for taking me to my first yoga class with Victor at the Shanti Yoga Ashram Center for Peace & Harmony, and to the most high for the continuous vibrant inspiration.

The Team

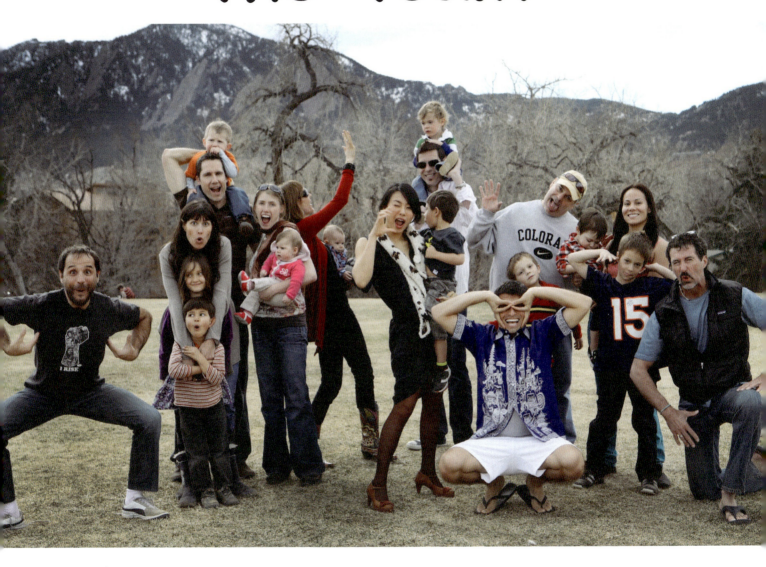

About the Author

Francisco has passion for healing, and yoga led him to new understandings of the human spirit and yogic practice. Traveling gives him the opportunity to work with amazing yogis from all over the world—especially yoga mamas who are forging new paths of understanding on the healing power of yoga during pregnancy.

Francisco's journey started with his work with conservation and cultural education projects across the United States with the National Audubon Society and the National Parks Conservation Association. During this time, he was able to work on keeping his mind and body liberated through the practice of Capoeira (a Brazilian martial art) and was introduced to Bikram yoga. The Bikram practice inspired him to leave his job and go to yoga training at the Shanti Yoga Center, Bikram Yoga Teacher Training, and Dharma Mittra.

Having a playful approach to yoga and zest for life led Francisco to create Synergy, which emphasizes the interconnection between themes of trust, connection, and playfulness. These connections are made through the art of partner stretching, Thai massage, and flying. Synergy workshops are held worldwide, attracting yogis from all walks of life. Visit www.synergy.com.pe to find out when the next journey is taking place.

Share your journey and practice with us by joining our community.
Like us on Facebook:
Facebook.com/PregnancyJourneyThroughYoga

Stay tuned for the next book communicating the art of Synergy
Visit us at:
SynergyPartnerYoga.com

Made in the USA
Charleston, SC
21 May 2014